This book will help the diabetic live with his condition on the best possible terms by providing him, his family, and his friends with a full understanding of the disease, the medical principles underlying its management, and the problems imposed and how they may be met.

How to Live with Diabetes

REVISED EDITION

HENRY DOLGER, M.D.
Chief, Diabetes Clinic, Mt. Sinai Hospital, New York

and **BERNARD SEEMAN**

 PYRAMID BOOKS   NEW YORK

HOW TO LIVE WITH DIABETES

A PYRAMID BOOK
Published by arrangement with W. W. Norton & Company, Inc.

Norton edition published 1958
Norton revised edition published 1965
Pyramid edition published October 1960
Pyramid revised edition published May 1966
    Second printing, October 1966
    Third printing, March 1967
    Fourth printing, August 1967
    Fifth printing, December 1967
    Sixth printing, April 1968
    Seventh printing, September 1968

PYRAMID BOOKS are published by Pyramid Publications, Inc.
444 Madison Avenue, New York, New York 10022, U.S.A.

Contents

PART ONE   The Disease

1   What About Diabetes? _____ 13
2   Who Gets Diabetes? _____ 21
3   The Development of Diabetes _____ 28
4   The Search for a Cure _____ 37

PART TWO   The Management of Diabetes

5   Diet and Diabetes _____ 49
6   The Meaning of Insulin _____ 61
7   Control with Insulin—the Tools _____ 71
8   Control with Insulin—the Techniques _____ 81
9   Orinase and the Oral Drugs _____ 90
10   The Complications of Diabetes _____ 106

PART THREE   The Problems of Diabetes

11   The Diabetic Child _____ 123
12   The Diabetic Adolescent _____ 138
13   The Diabetic Adult _____ 149
14   Diabetes as a Special Problem for Women ___ 160

PART FOUR   The Prospects

15   From Today to Tomorrow _____ 169
       Index _____ 185

Foreword

This is a book for diabetics and for those relatives and friends of diabetics whose lives may be touched by the disease.

Its major emphasis is on the person with diabetes rather than on the ailment or condition. While it deals with the questions of diagnosis and treatment, the book is more concerned with the human factors, the problems of daily living as they relate to growing up, work, marriage, sex, aging, and the means of adjusting to the numerous physical and emotional demands of the disease.

These matters are examined in detail and discussed realistically on the basis of day-by-day experience with thousands of diabetics of all ages.

In the main, attention is directed to those phases of the disease which the patient can help control. Certain complications which cannot be influenced by any direct contribution on the part of the diabetic are omitted.

This is no do-it-yourself manual and makes no effort to show the diabetic how to treat the disease on his own. Instead it is designed to help the reader understand diabetes on a medical as well as on a personal level. It deals with the medical aspects of the disease—its development, course and vagaries—so that the reader will be able to appreciate the principles behind the treatment prescribed by the physician and why sudden changes in treatment may be ordered.

The new oral drugs are discussed in detail; their characteristics, the areas in which they are useful, their modes of action insofar as these are known, and the dosage forms now available.

Also described are the newer concepts of diabetes as well as current research into the possible causes and the nature of the ailment, its detection prior to the appearance of overt symptoms (the "prediabetic" state) ; and the developing possibilties of diabetes prevention.

Since it is assumed that the diabetic is under medical care, the chapter on diets presents none of the currently used diet prescriptions. Where diets are used in treatment, they should be left to the judgment of the attending physician.

Altogether, the function of this book is to help the diabetic live with his disease. This requires the fullest possible understanding of the ailment, the medical principles underlying its management, the problems it imposes on the patient and his family and how these problems may be met.

Such an understanding should help arm the diabetic to face his disease on the best possible terms.

HENRY DOLGER, M.D.

New York, N.Y.

How to Live with Diabetes

PART ONE

The Disease

CHAPTER 1

What About Diabetes?

"Will I live?"

That is the first question a doctor usually hears when he tells a patient he has *diabetes mellitus*.

Then come other important questions.

"Will I be able to keep working?"

"Will I have to change my way of life?"

The answers are different today from what they would have been, say, in 1920. Given the benefits of modern treatment, the diabetic *can* live a normal life in virtually every respect. He can work, play, even be a parent. He can do almost everything the non-diabetic can do. But first, he must learn to live with his disease.

The diabetic should know everything that can be known about his ailment, its history, nature, how it develops, the problems it creates, how it is treated. He should understand the reasons for treatment. He should be able to distinguish medical fact from popular fancy, prejudice from sound practice. Knowing these things, he will be better able to cope with his disease every day of his life.

Diabetes mellitus is a metabolic disease. As far as we know, it is not caused by bacteria, viruses, or other microbes. It does involve an inability on the part of the body to perform certain vital functions. As a result, the diabetic is unable to use the carbohydrates he eats, the sugars and starches and turn them into the heat and energy his body needs to operate normally.

13

The Search for a Cause

Although diabetes is one of the oldest diseases known to man, its actual cause is unknown. Almost 3,500 years ago, a medical scribe of ancient Egypt described the disease in a manuscript now known as the Ebers Papyrus.

Physicians of ancient Greece also knew about this disease, and it was they who named it *diabetes* which means "siphon" in Greek. This refers to one of the most prominent symptoms of the ailment—frequent urination.

It was not until late in the seventeenth century that the adjective *mellitus* was added to the name to distinguish it from another disease named *diabetes insipidus. Mellitus* comes from the Latin word for honey and it refers to the fact that diabetics have sugar in their urine.

Early diagnosis involved tasting the urine. If it was sweet, the patient had *diabetes mellitus* and could expect about five to ten years more of life.

In 1783, an English physician, Thomas Cawley, became the first to record a diagnosis of *diabetes mellitus* by showing the actual presence of sugar in the urine. Five years later, while performing an autopsy, Cawley discovered an important clue to the possible cause of diabetes. He noticed that the pancreas, a gland just below and behind the stomach, seemed different in a diabetic than in a healthy person.

Cawley reported this observation but disregarded it himself since he was already convinced that diabetes was a disease of the kidneys. Perhaps if early records had been better kept or if scientific communication were on a more efficient level, Cawley would not have dismissed the importance of the pancreas. He might have known that in 1682 it had already been suggested that the pancreas was necessary for the complete utilization of carbohydrates.

Then, about 1860, Étienne Lancereaux, a Paris physician who had done considerable work with extremely emaciated diabetics, stated his conviction that diabetes *was* the result of a disordered pancreas.

The controversy continued to rage. While there were many theories about what started the disease, nothing very effective could be done to treat it, and the patients generally died. Still, reasoned the doctors, once the cause could be pinned down, the cure would logically follow.

A century after Thomas Cawley made his observation regarding a pancreatic change in a diabetic, two doctors performed an epoch-making experiment and stumbled upon an important fact as a result: In 1889, J. von Mering and O. Minkowski succeeded in removing the pancreas of a dog. In view of the fact that the dog survived the experiment, this was a remarkable feat.

Then the unexpected happened. The dog began to urinate with abnormal frequency, and clouds of flies gathered wherever he urinated. Bernhard Naunyn, von Mering's and Minkowski's medical superior, noticed this phenomenon and suggested that they analyze the dog's urine. They did and found that it contained sugar.

By removing the pancreas of the dog, the two doctors discovered that they had created a condition that duplicated diabetes in man. Step by step the diabetes symptoms developed until the animal passed into diabetic coma and died.

The discovery that removal of the pancreas resulted in diabetes did not produce a cure. So the search went on.

Meanwhile, a brilliant German medical student, Paul Langerhans, had made a remarkable advance. In the pancreas he found clusters of cells completely unlike the ordinary tissue of the gland. The purpose of these cells was still to be revealed, but they were given a somewhat romantic name—the islets of Langerhans.

Determined to find which part of the pancreas might be involved in diabetes, medical researchers continued their investigations. They tied up the main duct of the pancreas so that the gland shriveled, leaving only the islets of Langerhans intact. *This produced no diabetes.* But when the shriveled gland was removed *together with* the islets of Langerhans, *diabetes was produced.*

Was there something in the islets of Langerhans which made sugar metabolism possible—without which diabetes resulted?

It was while trying to find an answer to this question in 1921 that F. G. Banting and C. H. Best of Canada made their great discovery. It earned Banting a Nobel Prize and a knighthood, and gave the world the first effective means of treating diabetes.

The discovery was insulin, a hormone normally produced in the islets of Langerhans, which permits the body to metabolize sugars and starches and convert them into heat and energy.

The first human patient was a Toronto physician, Joe Gilchrist, who had severe diabetes. The results were described as "excellent."

Although the isolation of insulin provided a treatment for diabetes, it did not solve the problem of the underlying cause. Some people become diabetic even though their production of insulin is normal. Examination of diabetics killed in automobile accidents show some to have adequate concentrations of insulin in the pancreas.

Several Causes Seem Likely

In every case of diabetes there *does* seem to be some impairment of the insulin mechanism—either in its production or the way it works in the body. This has led scientists to suspect that what we know as *diabetes mellitus* may be several different diseases, each producing an inability to utilize carbohydrate due to insulin malfunction.

There are at least four factors which may interfere with normal insulin activity and thus produce diabetes:

1. There may be an inability to produce enough insulin because the pancreas is diseased or absent. Should the pancreas be damaged or destroyed by a tumor, or removed by surgery, diabetes invariably results.

2. There may be an increase in the rate at which the body uses up insulin. This may be caused by overeating or by overactivity of the thyroid gland. Where this creates an insulin shortage, diabetes results.

3. There may be an increase in the rate at which insulin is destroyed in the body. There may be a drop in insulin production, or its effects might be inhibited by the action of certain body chemicals. These chemicals include such enzymes as *insulinase* as well as insulin antibodies and certain proteins which attach themselves to insulin and inactivate it. In addition, the body may even produce abnormal insulin which is unable to fulfill its role in carbohydrate metabolism.

4. There may be a drop in the efficiency of insulin due to liver disease or the introduction into the system of certain chemicals which impede insulin activity. These chemicals include cortisone, ACTH, purified growth hormone as well as crude extracts of the pituitary gland. These might make the liver— the body's sugar storehouse—release more sugar into the blood than a normal insulin supply can handle.

5. In the alpha cells of the pancreas, the body produces a hormone which has an effect opposite to that of insulin. This substance is called *glucagon*, and it acts to release glucose from the liver into the blood. Normally, glucagon might thus help the individual survive during periods of starvation.

Any or all of these factors, as well as others not yet discovered, may bring about the set of symptoms we call *diabetes mellitus*. But the underlying cause or causes are still unknown. There are a number of theories but no conclusive proof.

Just as the cause of diabetes remains a mystery, so does the manner in which insulin works. Biochemists produce enough insulin to treat all diabetics who need it, but how this protein substance helps the body turn sugar into energy remains a puzzle.

At present there are three major theories, each of them involving complicated biochemical processes. One thing *is* certain about insulin, however. Scientists may not agree on *how* it works, but there is no disagreement about the fact that it *does* work, making it possible for a diabetic to live a fairly normal life.

But fairly normal does not mean perfectly normal. The diabetic faces hazards not common to the non-diabetic. There is a greater susceptibility to certain infections and ailments. There is a speeding-up of certain degenerative processes—especially in the eyes, kidneys, circulatory and nervous systems.

With proper care and careful hygiene some of these hazards may be controlled and held to a minimum. This must begin with prompt diagnosis—detecting the disease as soon at it appears.

The classical symptoms of diabetes, detailed in Chapter Three, are easy to recognize and show themselves in most, but not all, cases.

The majority of cases can be recognized readily enough by the physician, and while a few may present diagnostic problems, there is no reason why any diabetes should remain undetected and untreated.

The Meaning of Metabolism

Before we go any further into the details of diabetes, we should have a clear picture of what metabolism means to us. Unless we understand the metabolic process, the idea of a metabolic disease will be hard to grasp.

All of us must eat and breathe in order to live.

Eating provides us with nutrients such as carbohydrates, proteins, fats, minerals, and vitamins. Breathing provides us with oxygen.

The nutrients we eat and the oxygen we breathe are used by the body to make possible all the countless activities necessary to life.

Two fundamental processes are involved in metabolism. One is known as *anabolism*. The other is *catabolism*.

Anabolism means building up. The simple chemicals into which our foods have been reduced by digestion are rearranged and built into substances the body needs—new cells, tissues, blood, bone, muscle, and other material necessary to health and life.

Catabolism means breaking down. Worn-out or damaged cells and tissues of the body, materials that have served their purpose and are no longer needed, are broken down into simple chemicals. Depending upon the needs of the body, these may be eliminated as waste or rearranged and used again in some other form. In the various stages of catabolism, energy is released.

These two processes of metabolism are continuous whether we are at work or at rest, awake or asleep. But the tempo at which they operate keeps changing as the demands upon our bodies change with stress, activity, growth, illness, or aging.

For proper health there should be a balance between the foods we eat and the metabolic needs of the body.

If we eat too little food, the body turns upon itself and breaks down its own tissues—fats and proteins—to provide energy and chemicals for essential life functions. This is what happens when we go on weight-reducing diets. Carried to extremes, it results in starvation.

If we eat too much food, the excess is converted into fat which the body stores away. This results in overweight and obesity.

Our food needs and metabolic activity are highest in infancy, childhood, and adolescence, since that is when we have the greatest rate of growth. As we get older and stop growing, the food intake must be reduced to match the decreasing need.

With old age our energy needs decline, causing a progressive slowing of our metabolic tempo. So our food needs diminish further. This is why elderly people may put on excess weight although they eat no more than before.

By viewing metabolism as a continuous process that provides heat, energy, and living substance from the food we eat and the air we breathe, we can see that without metabolism there can be no life, and with faulty metabolism there can be no health.

When a person get *diabetes mellitus,* a very important part of the metabolic process breaks down. What happens as a result is similar to what happens in starvation, and many of the symptoms are the same.

Where the starving person can use carbohydrates but does not have them, the diabetic has them but cannot use them. The outcome is the same, but for one major difference. In the diabetic, the unused sugar piles up in the bloodstream and body tissues, then "spills" over into the urine. The kidneys work continuously to get rid of the excess sugar. This drags water out of the system and causes dehydration and insatiable thirst.

Since the body needs energy to live, and the usual foods do not provide it, the body begins to consume itself. This process, the same in diabetes as in starvation, is not very efficient in energy production. As it continues, dangerous by-products of fat metabolism are formed.

Known as ketone bodies or acetone, these chemicals are poisonous to the system in large quantities. They accumulate in the bloodstream, pour into the urine and, as the diabetic becomes less able to handle the rising ketone level, acidosis sets in. This is followed by coma and, finally, death.

That would be the course of diabetes if left untreated. And, before the isolation of insulin in 1921, diabetes was almost invariably fatal.

We have come a long way in the last few decades—more than the preceding thirty-five centuries. Diabetes may still be almost as much a mystery as it ever was, but it is no longer as big a problem.

This does not mean that diabetes is on the decline. It does mean that we are at last able to live with it. In view of the fact that more of us can expect to become diabetic as our life span increases, this represents substantial progress.

CHAPTER 2

Who Gets Diabetes?

Practically anybody can get diabetes, regardless of age, sex, race, or social station.

According to the latest estimates, some four million Americans currently have diabetes. Unlike polio, tuberculosis, and pneumonia it is not a disease that is on the wane. Instead it grows more prevalent as it reaches out to mark an increasing number of people each year.

About 200,000 Americans are diagnosed as diabetic each year according to a U.S. Government survey. This figure will increase as our population grows and becomes older.

What is more, during the next few decades the rate of increase in the number of diabetics in this country will be more than four times greater than the rate of increase in the total population.

The youngest diabetics ever recorded were a brother and sister. The girl became diabetic at the age of 4 months. Her infant brother was diagnosed as a diabetic at the age of 9 days. Today, almost ten years after the onset of the disease in the boy, both children receive small amounts of insulin daily and are growing normally.

Diabetes has been called a disease of old age. This is not strictly true. While 80 percent of all diabetics are over 40 years of age, there is also a considerable incidence of the disease in childhood, adolescence, and young adulthood.

The United States Public Health Service estimates that there are 1.7 diabetics for every 1,000 people up to age 24; 10.2 between the ages of 25 and 44; 33.1 per 1,000 in the 45 to 54 age group; 55.6 between ages 55 and 64; and 68.6 between 65 and 74.

In Britain, the Bedford Survey estimated that there are 200,000,000 diabetics in the world and that 14.5 percent of the individuals over age 50 are diabetic.

As far as age is concerned, we are susceptible to diabetes throughout our lifetimes. Our susceptibility increases gradually until we reach the age of 40. Then there is a rapid jump in susceptibility.

Females Are More Susceptible

Diabetes overlooks neither sex but it *does seem* to have a special preference for women. During childhood, adolescence, and young adulthood, the disease plays no favorites between the sexes. At the age of 30, the woman becomes more susceptible until, between 45 and 65, she is twice as likely as a man to get the disease. A striking increase in susceptibility occurs as the woman approaches the menopause.

One of the most unusual aspects of the disease is the apparent link to marriage and motherhood. The highest number of deaths from diabetes is among married women—and this includes widows and divorcées. The death rate among married women is almost twice as great as among single women.

The married man is far less susceptible than the married woman. For him, the wedded state acts as a protection, and his death rate from diabetes is lower than that of bachelors, widowers or divorcés.

Why should women be more susceptible to diabetes than men, and married women more than single women? Motherhood seems to be the reason. The woman with more children is more susceptible than the women with fewer children. The more pregnancies a woman undergoes, the greater is the possibility that she will become diabetic.

In 1949, three Scottish doctors, H. N. Munro, J. C. Eaton, and A. Glen, completed a thorough survey on the subject in a Glasgow Diabetes Clinic.

Obesity and heredity are ordinarily considered major factors in diabetes susceptibility. The increased susceptibility of married women has been attributed to the fact that they are frequently overweight during and after pregnancy.

To check this theory, the Scottish doctors studied a number of women of comparable obesity and found that the tendency toward diabetes varied directly with the number of children each woman had borne. The highest incidence was among the women with the biggest families.

As for the influence of heredity, the doctors found that women with six or more children were likely to get the disease even where there was no history of diabetes in the family.

These studies were conducted carefully to make a clear division between obesity and heredity on one hand, and frequency of motherhood on the other. The results showed that childbearing, by itself, must be considered an important factor in the development of diabetes among women.

Still another element in diabetes susceptibility is the size of the infant a woman bears. Not long ago—and in some areas even today—many parents fel that a bigger baby was a healthier baby. Today we know that an infant's size is no measure of its health, and the bigger the infant, the greater the likelihood that the mother will become diabetic. The woman who bears a child weighing ten pounds or more has a greater than 75 percent chance of becoming diabetic.

Thus, the reason for the sharp rise in diabetes among women over 40 seems mainly due to the stress of repeated pregnancy plus the dynamic upheaval of the menopause.

Race and Nationality Are Not Factors

A number of theories have linked diabetes to race, nationality, and geography. Negroes, for example, were supposed to have less diabetes than whites; Chinese and Japanese, less than Europeans.

The reason Southern Negroes appeared to have less diabetes was because they were less likely to have proper medical treatment, and less diabetes was therefore diagnosed.

In urban areas, where medical care and diagnosis are more easily available, existing diabetes is more frequently recognized and reported than in rural areas. These factors, not race or nationality account for, say, the apparently higher rate of diabetes among Jewish people, concentrated, as most are, in cities. And in the cities of the North diabetes is just as frequent among Negroes as among whites.

In areas where there is marked undernutrition and semi-starvation, there is less diabetes. In India, for instance, diabetes is not uncommon; but because of the low-calorie, low-protein, low-fat diet, the disease is usually mild. In the more prosperous, better-fed classes, however, diabetes seems to be more frequent and more severe.

The relationship between diabetes and what, how well, and how much we eat is remarkable. During the war, as food restrictions and rationing increased, the severity of existing diabetes decreased; the incidence of new cases declined.

Changing cultural and economic factors have their effect upon diet and stress patterns and thus also influence the incidence of diabetes. The Indians living and working in Natal, South Africa, have the highest diabetes rate in the world—42 percent of all adults.

This can also be seen among Yemenite Jews who, one decade after their arrival in Israel, showed a rise in diabetes incidence from practically zero to one half that of the Israelis of European origin.

Overeating and Diabetes

People who overeat are more susceptible to diabetes than those who do not. Where food intake is greater than the metabolic need, the possibility of diabetes increases. This is true regardless of race, nationality, geography, or whether one lives in the city or the country.

Because diabetes results from an inability to metabolize sugars, there is a popular belief that healthy people who eat excessive sweets tend to get diabetes. Yet some of the countries which have the highest sugar consumption seem to have lower diabetes records. On the other hand, the Natal Indians, working on sugar plantations and taking about 30 percent of their nourishment in sugar cane, have an exceptionally high diabetes rate.

Some researchers show that there *is* a relationship between the amount of fat in the diet and the tendency toward diabetes. But the really big dietary factor is not so much *what* you eat as *how much* you eat.

Plain overeating is today accepted as the most common precipitating factor in diabetes. This is not to imply that every overweight person—or even the majority of them—will become diabetic. But at least three of every four adults who became diabetic were overweight before they developed the disease.

Let us try to follow the process that may lead from overeating to diabetes.

As we eat more than we normally need, the pancreas has to produce additional insulin to handle the extra carbohydrates. The body can cope with this extra demand for insulin. But excess eating continues and the need for extra insulin increases to the point where production begins to fall behind the demand. When that happens, an *insulin deficiency* results. That is another way of saying diabetes has set in.

Since the insulin deficiency in this case exists only because of abnormal eating, reduction of weight and food intake can restore the metabolic balance and is usually enough to control the diabetes.

Heredity and Diabetes

If obesity is the most common *precipitating* factor in diabetes, heredity is the most important *predisposing* factor.

The influence of heredity is often a very elusive element. A diabetic may prove to a doctor that neither his parents, grandparents, nor great-grandparents had diabetes. This still would not eliminate the possibility of a hereditary predisposition. Many people who are latent diabetics may die from other causes *before* the disease develops. Children of these people may be predisposed to diabetes although their parents would seem to have been non-diabetic.

There is still another peculiarity about diabetic heredity. That is the factor called *anticipation*. When diabetes appears in a family it seems to develop earlier in each succeeding generation. The third generation gets it earlier in life than the second.

This may produce peculiar results in a long-lived family. A grandchild will become diabetic—to the amazement of all, since there is no family history of diabetes. Then the child's father or mother becomes diabetic. Finally the grandparent, the one who actually passed on the predisposition to the disease, is the last to be affected.

A final word about heredity. If we take the available facts into account, it would appear that in any tightly knit community or group where there is considerable inbreeding, the diabetes statistics are likely to go up.

There are several other factors in diabetes which should not be overlooked. Some ailments, particularly certain disturbances of the endocrine glands, may be responsible for an onset of diabetes.

Liver disease has been known to bring on diabetes by disturbing the body's sugar balance. Overactivity of the thyroid gland and the frontal lobe of the pituitary gland seem to influence our susceptibility.

Children who become diabetic are usually taller than average. This suggests a possible connection between juvenile diabetes and an excessive release of growth hormone from the anterior pituitary gland.

Victims of disease and various infections which produce great stress and shock, as well as people subjected to severe emotional upheavals, may find themselves somewhat more likely to develop diabetes. The likelihood is increased further if they have any inherent tendencies toward the disease.

Now let us return to the question asked at the head of this chapter:

Who Gets Diabetes?

Practically anybody can get diabetes, but an adult is more likely to get it than a child.

A person of a diabetic family is more likely to get it than a person of a non-diabetic family.

An overweight person is more likely to get it than a person of normal weight.

A person between the ages of 45 and 70 is more likely to get it than a person in any other age group.

An unmarried man is more likely to get it than a married man.

A woman is more likely to get it than a man.

A married woman is more likely to get it than an unmarried woman.

A mother is more likely to get it than a non-mother.

A mother of more children is more likely to get it than a mother of fewer children.

A mother of larger infants is more likely to get it than a mother of smaller infants.

On the basis of all this, the most likely candidates for diabetes are women between the ages of 45 and 70, who come from diabetic families and are overweight.

Of these, the greatest susceptibility of all lies with the mothers of many "king-sized" infants.

CHAPTER 3

The Development of Diabetes

The classical symptoms of diabetes are so obvious that it should be impossible to miss them. Yet too many people either are unaware of the signs or refuse to recognize them for what they are. The result—for every four known cases of diabetes, about three are undetected and untreated.

Here are the usual symptoms of diabetes in the approximate order they show themselves.

> Frequent, copious urination.
> Abnormal thirst.
> Rapid loss of weight.
> Extreme hunger.
> General weakness.
> Drowsiness and fatigue.
> Itching of the genitals and skin.
> Visual disturbances, blurring, etc.
> Skin disorders such as boils, carbuncles, and infections.

When these symptoms begin to appear, diabetes is not necessarily certain, but a trip to the doctor is clearly indicated.

Often, the classical symptoms do not show themselves. In those cases, some complication arises out of diabetes may provide the first clue. A kidney or circulatory disturbance, a stillbirth or other childbearing difficulty all may be signs of diabetes.

Diabetes varies with the people who have it. The severity and course of the illness may change from person to person; may even change within the same person as the result of some new experience.

Many factors influence the course of diabetes—illness, infection, emotional and physical stress, pregnancy. As a result, mild diabetes may suddenly become severe; stable diabetes may become unpredictable. In one case, loss of weight may seemingly eliminate the symptoms of the disease. In another case, a rapid loss of weight may be a sign that mild diabetes has abruptly turned severe.

With so many possible variations, it is not easy to classify the different degrees of diabetes. But some form of classification is necessary and, over a period of years, certain categories have been established. These must never be considered as final because time and the experiences of living may create changes in the diabetic and in the nature of his disease.

There are two common classifications of diabetes. The first is called *juvenile* or *insulin-deficient* diabetes. It is also known as *brittle* diabetes and accounts for about 30 percent of all cases.

The second category is *adult* or *maturity-onset* diabetes.

Each of these seems to have certain clear characteristics of its own. *Juvenile* diabetes is the form the disease takes in all diabetic youngsters and adolescents. *But it is not confined to juveniles.* Some adults get it; and a few adults suffering from the milder *maturity-onset* form may suddenly have their disease take a turn to the more severe juvenile or *insulin-deficient* form.

Characteristics of Childhood Diabetes

A fundamental difference between *juvenile* diabetes and *adult* diabetes is in the insulin situation. In *juvenile* diabetes there is an absolute deficiency of insulin. This means that the pancreas does not produce even the minimum of insulin needed for bare survival. Therefore, the insulin balance can only be brought to normal by making up the deficit through insulin injections.

With a few possible exceptions, all *juvenile* or *insulin-deficient* diabetics need insulin injections in order to live. On the other hand, many *adult* diabetics can manage their disease on diet alone.

There are also other differences. In *juvenile* diabetes, boys and girls are equally susceptible. Obesity is *not* a factor, as in *adult* diabetes. Instead, the juvenile patient is usually underweight when the disease strikes; he is also frequently taller than average.

In children, the onset of *juvenile* diabetes often seems very sudden. Actually, it may not be as sudden as it appears. The disease may have been developing at a slower, undetected rate, when, as is so frequent with children, mumps, measles, chickenpox or one of the other ailments of childhood steps in. Then, as a result of this other ailment, the diabetes flares up dramatically, seeming to appear out of nowhere.

In children and adolescents especially, *juvenile* diabetes is very unstable. The patient's need for different insulin dosages shifts unpredictably as his blood-sugar levels undergo wide fluctuations. This is due to the fact that the demands of growth impose a need for constantly increasing calorie intake and for more carbohydrates.

Children are also more likely than adults to subject their bodies to greater extremes of physical activity— with more violent bursts of exertion on the one hand and longer periods of sleep on the other.

The diabetic child needs insulin injections from the start of the disease, and the dosage usually increases progressively as the child grows older. When adulthood is reached, the dose becomes relatively stable.

There is one more important characteristic of *juvenile* diabetes—a distinct sensitivity to insulin. The *juvenile* or *insulin-deficient* diabetic responds very sharply to its absence or presence. Too little insulin may bring about an abrupt rise in blood-sugar. Slightly too much insulin may cause too rapid a drop in blood-sugar and bring on an insulin reaction.

Characteristics of Adult Diabetes

The characteristics of *adult* or *maturity-onset* diabetes are quite different from the *juvenile* form. The overwhelming majority of diabetics—some 70 percent —are adults who do not acquire the disease until they have passed the age of 35. Most of them are overweight when the disease strikes.

This form of diabetes usually results from a relative

rather than an absolute insufficiency of insulin as in
juvenile diabetes. The *maturity-onset* diabetic need
not have a flagrant lack of insulin. He may even have
an ordinarily normal insulin supply. But, because
something impedes the action of his insulin supply, he
gets less insulin activity than he needs for proper carbohydrate metabolism.

Adult diabetes may be mild, moderate, or severe, depending upon the amount of insulin needed to keep it
under control. About half of the cases are classified as
mild and do not require insulin injections. These can
usually be treated with relatively mild dietary restrictions.

There are a number of overweight diabetics whose
insulin production is normal but who overeat to the
point where they take in more carbohydrate than their
insulin supply can cope with. In many such cases, a return to normal weight is enough to correct the relative
insufficiency of insulin and free the patient from the
symptoms of diabetes.

About half of the adult diabetics may be of normal
weight. They do not overeat to any great extent but
they do, for some reason or other, have something
wrong with the way their insulin works.

If there is a ten percent impairment of insulin function, this can be equalized by a ten percent reduction
in dietary carbohydrate. But if the drop in insulin
efficiency is greater than ten percent, additional food
reduction would cause underweight, loss of strength
and a decline in working ability. Therefore insulin injections or Orinase, or other new drugs which can be
taken by mouth, are needed.

All this may seem very cut-and-dried. But even
adult diabetes, usually more predictable than *juvenile*
diabetes, has its surprises.

Take an obese individual who constantly overeats.
In order to handle his excess carbohydrates, his pancreas becomes overactive and produces more than the
normal amount of insulin. If there is no inherent susceptibility and no great stress, he may go on all his

life and never develop diabetes.

On the other hand, if he has a diabetic heredity or if he encounters some great physical or emotional stress, a relative insulin shortage may result. The pancreas, though still healthy, cannot produce that extra amount of needed insulin. A diet, reducing the obesity and cutting the excess carbohydrate, may restore the balance and remove the diabetes symptoms.

Suppose this same person who develops a relative insulin shortage does not treat it, or while treating it, suffers a prolonged illness or other stress. This may cause the insulin-producing cells of his pancreas to overwork, give out, and atrophy, producing an *absolute* instead of a *relative* insulin shortage. In such cases we see obese adult diabetics developing the more severe *juvenile* or *insulin-deficient* diabetes.

Apart from their different characteristics, the two types of diabetes also develop differently.

How Juvenile Diabetes Develops

Juvenile diabetes, when it develops in childhood, should be relatively easy to recognize. Most often it begins with the classical symptoms. Where it is not promptly recognized, the error usually lies with the parents who are either unaware of medical developments or do not have an emotional acceptance of the child.

Bed-wetting is usually the first clue to diabetes in a child. Unfortunately, many parents simply regard this as a behavior disorder which they frequently punish.

The next clue is an insatiable thirst which cannot be quenched even with large quantities of soda pop, water and other fluids.

Then comes extreme hunger and weight loss. Growing children should be hungry. But when their normal hunger is intensified, and *they lose instead of gain weight,* the hunger may be caused by diabetes rather than the demands of growth.

By this time, with bed-wetting, thirst, hunger, and weight loss, the parents should certainly be aware that something is wrong with the child and that an immediate consultation with the doctor is necessary. Altogether too many children are not recognized as diabetic until the disease has become so severe that the young victims are in diabetic coma and need to be hospitalized.

Juvenile diabetics usually have a difficult and complicated problem. The younger the case, the greater and more exacting is the care needed to control the ailment.

Episodes of ketosis and coma are more frequent and more sudden in children because of their lower carbohydrate reserves. And, because of the inexorable demands of growth, children cannot accept food reductions as a treatment. For them, insulin is imperative.

Diabetic youngsters sometimes show a temporary remission of symptoms after the start of therapy. This may last for several months. But the need for insulin invariably returns and, with the rare exceptions where a change to an oral drug is possible, remains permanent.

As the diabetic child grows older and reaches adolescence, emotional disturbances related to the disease are often likely to arise. Various things are involved here—the tyranny of daily insulin injections, the need to eat at rigidly fixed times, the restrictions against candy and other sweets which their non-diabetic friends are free to enjoy, anxiety regarding too much physical activity (which may bring on insulin shock) or too little (which may bring on diabetic coma).

These and other factors arising out of his "difference" from other children—if they are emphasized—may add to the tensions and stress of the diabetic child. This, in turn, may stir up the basic instability of the disease and increase its severity.

As treatment of the disease improves, and enlightenment and understanding grows, more and more juvenile diabetics become adult men and women, carry on active and productive lives, marry and rear families. Measure this against the days before insulin when the juvenile diabetic was doomed to die within two years after the onset of the disease.

How Adult Diabetes Develops

The development of *adult* or *maturity-onset* diabetes is usually less severe and less sudden than *juvenile* diabetes. Also it is usually more difficult to detect.

The disease is often so mild at the outset that the patient may learn of it for the first time during a routine examination required by an insurance company for a policy. As a matter of fact, over 30 percent of *adult* diabetes is discovered in this casual way.

A man feels thirsty and starts drinking large quantities of liquids. He might attribute his thirst to the heat, the fact that he is working hard, or the fact that he is urinating a lot. On the other hand, his frequent urination may be attributed to the fact that he is doing a lot of drinking. So the symptoms of thirst and excessive urination may not be recognized for what they are.

Extreme hunger and loss of weight are obvious symptoms only in a minority of adults. Diabetes can and has developed in obese people while they were reducing. The loss of poundage is often gratefully accepted as being due to the reducing effort rather than to the diabetes.

All these and other factors frequently delay the recognition of diabetes in adults. The first clue to the presence of the disease may come as the result of a complication rather than from the diabetes itself.

During World War II, a young American lieutenant advancing through Germany attributed his thirst to the summer heat, and his frequent urination to the enormous quantities of beer he quaffed. But one day he became aware that his sexual urges were almost gone. This promptly brought him to the doctor and it was there that the diabetes was discovered.

Quite a number of patients may first go to a dentist because their teeth loosen or their gums became painful or abscessed. Others may go to a urologist because they think their excessive urination is due to a bladder or kidney infection. Some adults, worried about blurring vision, may go to an oculist. Women, perturbed about a persistent genital itch, may go to a gynecologist.

In all of these cases it may then be discovered that the obvious disorders are the result of diabetes.

Women may first become aware of diabetes during a pregnancy or after a stillbirth. Circulatory, kidney, skin, and other ailments may drive an adult to seek medical advice and so first become aware of the fact that he has diabetes.

There is still a further peculiarity of diabetes which can make it even more complicated and unpredictable than it normally is.

Let us imagine an adult with an inherent susceptibility to diabetes. Under ordinary circumstances, he may not develop his diabetes until he reaches the age of 50. But he has an automobile accident, he contracts a severe infection, his wife divorces him, he loses his job.

Under the impact of a series of stresses, his diabetes arrives at the age of 30. Then, as treatment is begun and takes hold, there may be an abrupt remission. The diabetes will mysteriously vanish, not to appear again until the age of 50 or thereabouts, when it orginally may have been due.

Situations like this do not happen often, but they *do* occur. For some susceptible people, the boat of their lives has to be rocked violently to bring on the symptoms of the disease. For others, the diabetes develops progressively.

Once the adult knows he has diabetes and treatment is begun, the chances are that he can live a relatively normal life. The aim of modern medicine is to make the disease and its treatment as inconspicuous as possible so that its intrusion on everyday living can be kept to a minimum. But the diabetic still must take some extra care of himself.

Young or old, he should try to live a regular life. He should try to keep his weight as nearly normal as possible. If he is being treated by diet alone, he should observe its limitations. If he is insulin-treated, his dosage, food intake, and energy output are all balanced. If any one of these is disturbed, he should rectify the others in order to maintain the balance. If he is orally treated, he may have greater flexibility but should still avoid any excess.

The diabetic who is able to keep all these factors under control will still remain diabetic for the rest of his life; but he will be able to function every bit as well as the non-diabetic and live as fully.

Some of the world's most noted figures have been diabetic. Among them, writer-historian H. G. Wells, novelist Hugh Walpole, statesman Georges Clemenceau, artist Paul Cézanne, composer Giacomo Puccini, and political leader Fiorello H. LaGuardia all lived full and productive lives. Athletic prominence, too, has been achieved by diabetics. Notable here is tennis star Billy Talbert, who represented the United States on the Davis Cup team.

CHAPTER 4

The Search for a Cure

The search for a cure for diabetes has been one of the longest quests in the history of the human race.

It began some 3,500 years ago, perhaps a century before Moses led the Israelites out of Egypt, and to this day the cure is still beyond our reach.

We *have* made progress, but basically all that we have achieved, and that relatively recently, is a means of treating the major symptom of diabetes—the inability to metabolize sugar.

The diabetic cannot be cured of his disease as he might be cured of measles, diphtheria, pneumonia, or jaundice. But he can be treated so that the effects are reduced and the disease itself, while not erased, is kept under control.

This does not imply that a cure cannot or will not be found. But the great problem facing medical researchers has been the fact that they still do not know the cause or causes of the disease. They only know its intermediate effect—that something goes wrong with the insulin mechanism, thus interfering with carbohydrate metabolism.

Curing diabetes or any other disease generally involves knowing and eliminating the cause. There are cases where cures have been stumbled upon before the cause of a disease was known. This may result from a happy accident or after many generations of trial and error. The English were able to cure and prevent scurvy by including citrus fruits in the diet long before it was discovered that Vitamin C existed or that scurvy was due to a deficiency of this vitamin.

Lucky events like these are rare and, as far as diabetes is concerned, the disease appears much too complicated to be tracked down to a single cause. Many factors are involved—the pancreas, the liver, and the ductless glands such as the thyroid, adrenal, and pituitary. But in all cases the result is approximately the same. Whatever the cause, insulin action is impaired and that, at least, can be treated.

Treatments and even "cures" have almost always existed. But none of these "cures" worked and, until recently, neither did the treatments.

The Ebers Papyrus, which dates from about 1,500 B.C., is one of the oldest of all medical documents. It came into the hands of George Ebers in Luxor, Egypt, in 1872 and was completely translated in 1890.

From this manuscript it appears that the physicians of ancient Egypt had at least four "cures" for diabetes. The prescriptions were listed under the following heading:

"A medicine to drive away the passing of too much urine."

Typical of these earliest "cures" was the first one listed in the manuscript:

Prescription:

	Cakes	
Fresh grits	1/8
Wheat grains	1/8
Green lead earth	1/8
Water	1/3

Let stand moist; strain it; take it for four days.

How the Egyptian patients fared under these "cures" is not known. Certainly they were not cured.

Early Description of the Disease

In the second century of the Christian era, a truly remarkable physician known as Aretaeus the Cappadocian—Cappadocia was the name of a mountainous region near the Euphrates River in what is now Turkey—gave an astonishingly accurate account of the disease.

"Diabetes," he wrote, "is a wonderful affection, not very frequent among men, being a melting down of the flesh and limbs into urine . . ."

He went on to describe most of the symptoms and then made a speculation as to the cause.

"The cause of it may be that some one of the acute diseases may have terminated in this . . ."

Today's scientists have pretty much gone back to a similar view—that diabetes does not have a single direct origin but that it results, instead, from other disturbances in the body.

Another "cure" for diabetes was advanced in the

sixteenth century by a physician with the improbable name of Theophrastus Bombastus von Hohenheim. Known as [Philippus Aureolus] Paracelsus, he is recognized today as one of the medical giants of history, with views far in advance of his time.

According to Paracelsus, diabetes was due to the accumulation of a salt in the system. To cure it, he suggested fasting for two days, drinking "Julep" to relieve the thirst and getting rid of the salt.

The years passed. Men and women continued to become diabetic and, whether they remained untreated or whether they took the then-accepted "cure," there was little difference in the outcome. They died, usually within five years after the onset of the disease.

It remained for an English physician of the seventeenth century, Thomas Willis, to bring a measure of scientific sanity to the search for a diabetes cure. Willis, a man possessing great powers of clinical observation, took the trouble to taste the urine of diabetics and described it as "wonderfully sweet as it were imbued with Honey or Sugar."

In a book published in London in 1679, Willis wrote that "it seems a most hard thing in this Disease to draw propositions for curing for that its cause lies so deeply hid . . ."

So a circle was completed and the disease which could not be cured by the Egyptians—although they thought they had several cures—still could not be cured after several thousand years of observation and countless so-called remedies.

The First Real Dietary Treatment

It was not until 1796 that the first rational attempt was made at the treatment of diabetes through diet. This was an epoch-making step since it did not pretend to cure the ailment, but sought to make it possible for the diabetic to live with his disease.

Oddly enough, the advance was made by a military physician, John Rollo, surgeon general of the British Royal Artillery. Although the science of nutrition had not yet advanced to the point where proteins, carbohydrates, and the other nutrients were properly recognized—let alone classified and understood—the Rollo diet seemed to avoid carbohydrates in favor of proteins. The diet was, said Rollo, "to consist of animal foods principally."

Despite many shortcomings, the dietary approach opened by Rollo raised the curtain on what was to be —until the isolation of insulin—the first effective means of *treating* diabetes. Until 1922, when insulin replacement became a new basis for treatment, *diet formed the only useful approach to diabetes care*.

The great majority of diets emphasized deprivation. Some patients were helped by some diets, others were injured. Good or bad, each diet had its zealous disciples who maintained that theirs was the only true way and that the others were, at best, mistaken—at worst, a deadly heresy.

At one time, diabetics were made to drink their own urine as a means of restoring lost sugar. In 1857, P. A. Piorry of France fed his diabetic patients more than a quarter of a pound of candy daily to compensate for the loss of sugar through the urine.

Over a period of years, the treatment of diabetics took on the overtones usually associated with the primitive religious ritual of "mortification of the flesh" as a sort of penance of original sin. Only in this case the sin consisted of being a diabetic.

There can be no question that diet saved many lives. This is particularly true of the diet evolved by F. M. Allen in 1914. The Allen diet involved total restriction of calories and emphasized vegetables cooked in three water changes, bran, and olive oil.

The hardships imposed by such a diet were pathetically illustrated by an emaciated 12-year-old boy, who surreptitiously ate his toothpaste and the birdseed of his pet canary.

The dawn of the insulin era, which provided the first original advance in the treatment of diabetes since the Pharaohs, made it possible to free many diabetics from the dietary rigors imposed by earlier treatments. It permitted the use of a higher carbohydrate intake and released millions of diabetics from the often ritualized masochism of self-denial. It also made possible a longer and more normal life expectancy for the diabetic. *But it is not a cure.*

Insulin injections only treat a symptom of diabetes. This is the absence or inactivity of the normal insulin we need to help us metabolize sugars. The injected insulin replaces the absent insulin or reinforces the inactive insulin, but it does not touch the cause of diabetes. Therefore insulin injections are not the perfect answer except in the rare cases where the patient's pancreas is destroyed or has been removed by surgery.

Doctors Differ over Treatment

Although the search for a cure has been held back by the delay in finding the fundamental causes of the disease, there is still another impediment—the fanaticism which has developed around the various approaches to treatment.

Insulin did, after all, free the diabetic from the rigors of a diet that often caused unnatural hardship. Yet, not only were there some who refused to ease the rigidity of the diet, but there is still sharp division over the choice of diet and the type of insulin that should be used. There is even disagreement as to the goals that treatment should seek to accomplish.

One group of doctors holds that the first object of treatment is to keep the urine free of sugar. This is a traditional approach and has a large, influential following.

Another group of diabetes specialists takes a somewhat different view. They feel it is rarely practical to keep the urine constantly free of sugar because this may require a diet that would make it impossible for the diabetic to share in the normal enjoyment of living. Furthermore, they say, overemphasis of this objective of treatment often saddles the patient with worry, depression, inconvenience, and a sense of guilt.

The doctors who support the second viewpoint feel that the important thing in the insulin-treated patient is to keep the sugar level of the blood within bounds, and that moderate amounts of urinary sugar should not cause undue worry. They hold that modern therapy has reduced the need for a rigid diet since, with insulin, the diabetic *can* metabolize carbohydrates. Furthermore, in most cases the insulin dosage can be adjusted to allow the patient to devote more time to enjoying his meals and less time to worrying about them.

Of course, even these doctors agree that some dietary restriction is necessary, especially in obese patients and where there are complications.

The average diabetic, as he views the extremes of this controversy, might well ask himself:

Did the discovery and isolation of insulin free me from slavery to a diet? Or did it merely add the new inconvenience of insulin injections to the existing hardships of the diet?

The truth is that old habits die very hard, particularly if these habits have become fixed and enshrined.

As with any new treatment, insulin came in for sharp scientific scrutiny and considerable resistance on the part of doctors who wanted to be sure that the insulin worked and that the possible harm it might do did not outweigh the potential benefits. This is all part of a normal and natural process. Too much is at stake—human life—to permit acceptance of anything new without substantial proof of its safety and efficacy.

But insulin ran into a further obstacle, the resistance of the "diet-only" cult of treatment. Then, as insulin established itself as the basis of diabetes treatment, the cultists began to accept it and even developed a new cult around it.

Thus, the inflexible ritual of the daily insulin injection, the veneration of sugar-free urine, the dietary taboos and the sense of sinful guilt on the taking of "forbidden sweets" all became part of the new religious discipline of diabetes treatment. And the physician remained vested with the power to reward the patient with an extra slice of bread or to impose the "penance" of additional dietary restrictions.

Pediatricians Force Easing of Rigid Diet

The first break in the "rigid diet" front came in the 1930s as a result, oddly enough, of the pressure of pediatricians. With insulin already in use more than ten years at the time, pediatricians found that diabetic youngsters still did not grow well as a result of undernourishment. Although they were receiving insulin to help them metabolize sugars, they were not being allowed diets to satisfy the caloric needs of growing children.

The pediatricians began to exert pressure to improve the children's diets, urging a more normal caloric intake. The use of insulin, they maintained, had made dietary improvement possible and there was no longer any reason to cling to unnecessary and even dangerous restrictions.

Under this pressure the diets were modified. Gradually the feeling grew and spread that the diabetic—even the adult diabetic—could be allowed to enjoy more normal nutrition as a consequence of insulin.

Today, while the dietary situation has improved considerably, there is still some resistance to change and the tug of war goes on.

The search for a cure did not end with insulin's isolation—although the hormone is so effective a treatment that, for a time, new research lost a good deal of its urgency. But insulin is not a cure, nor is it the perfect treatment. Some patients resist insulin and need unusually large amounts. It has to be handled carefully and administered in exact dosages. Furthermore, while it may free the diabetic from the unyielding adherence to a rigid diet, it also chains him to the need for daily insulin injections and exposes him to the hazards of insulin shock.

The fact that insulin has to be injected has been a major problem. Since it is a protein substance, it is destroyed by the digestive juices and therefore cannot be taken by mouth. This creates a number of special problems. The diabetic, obviously, cannot be expected to go to his doctor every day for his injection. Consequently he must give it to himself or have some relative or neighbor give it to him. It is easy to see how the need for insulin injections, apart from being inconvenient, may sometimes become a distinct hardship.

So, from the very moment insulin was discovered, a search was begun for a drug which could be taken by mouth to control diabetes.

In June, 1957, after an intensive period of work which had been set into motion as the result of a series of medical accidents, the first substance which could be taken by mouth to reduce blood sugar was released to physicians in the United States. The drug, already widely used in Europe, has the chemical name of tolbutamide and is distributed in this country and Canada as Orinase. In the rest of the world it is known as Rastinon.

Although it is a thoroughly tested drug, Orinase has met with some resistance, as did insulin in its day. Much of this arises from the fact that the way in which the drug works is not yet known.

Ordinarily, this is a valid scientific reason, since there is always a possibility that the unknown may be dangerous. Nevertheless, understanding the mode of action of a useful drug is not always a guarantee of safety, nor is absence of understanding necessarily a bar to a drug's use. We still do not understand how insulin works, how many of the antibiotics work, or even how aspirin works.

While this oral drug is certainly no cure, it can replace insulin injections in many adult diabetics.

Even more important from a scentific standpoint, Orinase and the other oral drugs such as Diabinese, Dymelor, and DBI are providing a new surge of inspiration to diabetes investigation. Using these drugs as research tools, scientists have set into motion a tide of fresh investigation.

What they find most fascinating is the possibility that these drugs may help provide the key to the mystery of how insulin works. And this, in its turn, may open the long-locked door to the causes of diabetes and thus, after 3,500 years, bring within reach the possibility of a cure.

Another major advance toward the understanding of diabetes has been the synthesis of the insulin molecule.

In 1960, working independently, a Toronto group under G. H. Dixon and a Shanghai group under Y. C. Du split the insulin molecule into its component parts and then reconstituted it.

Following this achievement, a Pittsburgh team headed by P. G. Katsoyannis completely synthesized the separate A- and B-chains which, together, constitute the insulin molecule. These two chains were then linked by Dixon to form the complete hormone.

This was the first time so complex a molecule as insulin had been constructed by man. The importance of this accomplishment is almost beyond estimation at this time. It makes possible the creation of insulin with built-in radioactive tracers that may provide definitive clues as to precisely where and how this hormone achieves its metabolic effect. It also opens the way to the possible manipulation of the insulin molecule so that forms might be created that could be taken by mouth rather than by injection.

PART TWO

The Management of Diabetes

CHAPTER 5

Diet and Diabetes

Fifty years ago, the average diabetic faced a gloomy prospect. In severe cases, he usually died after a relatively short illness. In milder cases, he had the choice of a slightly longer life—perhaps five or more years—or, if he were willing to undergo the rigid deprivation of the existing treatment, possibly ten years of something less than life.

Today, with insulin, the new oral drugs, and better general treatment, a diabetic can enjoy a virtually normal life span. The doctor's goal in treating him is not merely to keep him alive but to make it possible for him to live, work, and function as fully as his capabilities permit.

The change that has taken place can be summed up by the catechism for diabetics developed by E. P. Joslin of Boston.

Prior to 1922, the question "What are you to do with an apple?" was to be answered, "give it away." Now, Joslin could accept the reply, "Eat it."

Difficult as the early treatments were for diabetics, the fact remains that they were treatments. They were hard on the patient—sometimes unbearable—but in many cases they permitted him to survive longer than would otherwise have been possible.

We have already noted that the first effective dietary approach came in 1796 when John Rollo undertook the treatment of a certain Captain Meredith. The treatment was rigorous, to put it mildly. In view of what the good captain underwent, he deserves almost as much credit for his fortitude as Dr. Rollo does for his superb medical achievement.

Captain Meredith's ordeal began with a bleeding; then, confined to a room, he was placed on the following diet:

"Breakfast, 1½ pints of milk and ½ pint of lime water mixed together; and bread and butter. For noon, plain blood puddings made of blood and suet only. Dinner, game or old meats which have been long kept; and as far as the stomach may bear, fat and rancid old meats, as pork. To eat in moderation. Supper, the same as breakfast."

In addition to this diet, Captain Meredith had his skin greased daily with lard; and an ulceration, the size of a half-crown, was maintained opposite each kidney.

The captain was 34 at the time and his diabetes, which had developed seven months earlier, was moderate. He improved steadily and, as his urine became sugar-free, the strict diet was gradually relaxed to include such vegetables as cabbage, lettuce, boiled onions, and radishes. In due time, Captain Meredith was able to resume his military career.

Early Diets Made Eating Loathsome

Rollo knew nothing of the metabolic nature of diabetes and the fact that it involves a failure of carbohydrate utilization. His diet, based on trial and error with a good helping of intuition, was truly a remarkable advance. In fact, some of the scientifically founded diets of the twentieth century were modifications of the Rollo diet which emphasized proteins and fats, curbed carbohydrates. It also curbed the total intake of food by making eating as distasteful as possible.

An insight into the theory behind this can be had from Dr. Rollo's account of two diabetics who, after consuming the lees of oil and drinking melted fat, "contracted so great a loathing of food, that neither of them ate anything for five days, and so got rid of their distempers."

The practice of curbing food intake by making eating unpleasant gathered great vogue in the years following the introduction of the Rollo diet.

Robert Watt of Scotland was one of a number of physicians who gave their patients antimony powders to curb their appetites. The powders, wrote Dr. Watt, "produced very severe sickness, vomiting, and commotion in the stomach and bowels. Anything which produces sickness has a temporary effect in relieving diabetes. . . ."

As the years passed, the strict animal diet with its emphasis on rancidity gradually changed. Apollinaire Bouchardat, one of the great diabetes clinicians of the last century, modernized the Rollo diet. He insisted on individualizing the treatment for each patient, objected to the rancidity of Rollo's fats and substituted fat and alcohol for carbohydrates.

Alcohol, since it requires no insulin, is readily converted into energy and was frequently used to replace carbohydrates in the diet of diabetics.

It was Bouchardat who began the practice of fastdays for diabetics. While he was the first to show the value of the intelligent use of exercise, he injected a religious quality into treatment by telling a patient who asked for bread, "You shall earn your bread by the sweat of your brow."

And the bread which he did allow had to be charred almost to a cinder before he permitted it to be eaten.

Most of the diets of the pre-insulin area were so harsh and restrictive that they were almost impossible to follow. The patients, being human, broke them with enough regularity to impede the treatment. Against this background came the Italian physician, Arnoldo Cantani, who practiced in the second half of the nineteenth century.

Dr. Cantani permitted his patients only lean meat and various fats. In milder cases, eggs, liver, and shellfish were allowed. The total food intake was strictly limited. Cantani felt that about a pound of cooked meat a day was all the food a diabetic needed.

In addition to this, if the urine still contained sugar, the patient had to fast as often as once a week. To make absolutely sure that his patients observed the diet he prescribed, Cantani took the precaution of imprisoning them in locked rooms.

The regular course of the Cantani treatment took three months. If the urine was not sugar-free in that time, the treatment was extended to six and even nine months.

By this time, various dietary schools had come into being, each upholding its particular approach with fierce partisanship. Men like Cantani and his German follower, Bernhard Naunyn, were champions of the rigid carbohyrate-free diet. On the other extreme were the high-carbohydrate schools. These included exponents of milk diets, cereal diets, potato diets, oatmeal diets and a number of others.

By the early part of this century, the partisanship was so intense that some physicians were arguing over the superiority of different brands of oatmeal and the various ways of cooking them.

Science vs. Dogmatism

As these controversies boiled, Naunyn gradually swung away from the extreme Cantani school and developed a diet more closely keyed to the caloric needs and tolerances of the individual patients. But the fast days persisted.

It remained for von Noorden, an eminent diabetes specialist of the era just before insulin, to label these fast days "metabolic Sundays," thus endowing them with an aura of religious self-denial.

Amid all the dogmatism, contradiction and confusion, there were a number of scientists who, instead of upholding this or that diet, were trying to learn more about diabetes.

Notable among these was Rudolph Eduart Külz, whose experiments uncovered many errors and superstitions then prevalent among doctors. In 25 years of clinical practice, Külz—who died in 1895 at the age of 50—made a careful study of 1,100 diabetics. Among other things, his experiments showed that a number of drugs widely used to reduce urinary sugar were not only useless but actually harmful. Furthermore, he demonstrated that mineral water had no effect on diabetes. This exploded a delusion that had made diabetics swarm to mineral springs as though they were shrines.

Some of Külz's most important work was in testing the tolerances of diabetics for various forms of carbohydrates. He found that diabetics assimilated starch from green vegetables better than from other sources, that certain forms of sugar—under certain circumstances—were better-assimilated than other forms.

In treating his patients, Külz resorted to neither undernutrition nor fasting. Instead, after testing the amount and kind of carbohydrate each patient could best tolerate, he worked out individualized diets to meet his patient's caloric needs.

While Külz and several other physicians were trying to work out rational approaches to diabetes treatment and were subjecting them to close scientific scrutiny, other doctors went their way enthusiastically promoting their pet panaceas.

The way some of these treatments were worked out was haphazard in the extreme. The one developed by Guelpa of Paris is a prime example.

The Guelpa treatment was born out of a medical error. A doctor studying the course of typhoid fever made a mistaken observation to the effect that "the more regular and rapid the patient's loss of weight" up to the disappearance of fever, "the quicker and more favorable was his course of recovery."

Although this later proved to be completely wrong, Guelpa seized upon it and applied it first to infections, then to diabetes. His sovereign remedy was to turn the patient into a living skeleton as quickly as possible.

In Guelpa's own words, " . . . the more promptly emaciation sets in, and the more definitely it establishes itself, the more sure and rapid is the patient's progress toward recovery."

To achieve this prompt emaciation, Guelpa subjected his patients to a series of three- to five-day fasts, during which they were copiously purged with cathartics. Between the fasting-purgation periods, the patients were allowed a week to a fortnight of carefully restricted diet which, for the first week, consisted of no more than 2½ pints of milk daily.

This technique of starving and purging patients to the point of emaciation was not confined to the treatment of diabetes. It was also recommended for gout, asthma, rheumatism, anemia, eczema, nervous disorders, insanity, epilepsy, drug addiction and a number of other afflictions. All this was not a product of the Middle Ages, but part of serious medical practice as late as 1911 and after.

There is even recorded a case, not treated by Guelpa, of an incipient diabetic who fasted for 20 days until his urine became sugar-free.

The Guelpa treatment succeeded in gaining some followers in England and France, and a few favorable results were observed among obese patients suffering from mild diabetes. But in cases of even moderate severity, the treatment was most likely to prove disastrous.

Diabetics Resist Extreme Diets

The normal urge to eat usually conflicted with the treatment. Even patients who willingly accepted restrictive diets—and this included undernutrition treatments less extreme than Dr. Guelpa's—soon found the self-deprivation unendurable. Unless they were locked away or under constant control, they lapsed from the "permitted" to the "forbidden."

A French physician, visiting the United States only a few years before the isolation of insulin, reported that in his country the patients were less willing than those in other countries to accept restrictive diets. Instead, he said, they wanted a diabetes treatment that would permit them to eat freely.

Like the great Athenian orator, Demosthenes, diabetics complained of "the diet prescribed by doctors, which neither restores the strength of the patient nor allows him to succumb."

As more was learned about diabetes, attempts were made to regulate the food intake so that the patient would neither accumulate excess sugar in the system nor toxic amounts of ketone and acetone. These are the metabolic by-products when fat and protein are substituted for carbohydrates as an energy source. Patients on the verge of coma from excess ketone and acetone were taken off fats and proteins and put on a limited carbohydrate diet. When their urinary sugar rose dangerously they were taken off carbohydrates and put on fats and proteins.

This dietary juggling had to be closely controlled in order to adjust for any metabolic fluctuations that might arise. In mild cases, and even in some moderate cases where the patient was obese, diet could be helpful if for no other reason than that it curbed overeating and overweight. In a number of cases this was able to reduce the patient's food intake to the point where his limited natural insulin supply no longer faced more work than it could handle.

As a result of dietary improvement, the rise in the life expectancy of diabetics was not very great but at least it was measurable.

Herbert H. Marks of the Metropolitan Life Insurance Company, one of the nation's foremost medical statisticians, has shown from the experience of the George F. Baker Clinic in Boston, that during what is known as the era of the Naunyn diet—1897 to 1914—

a ten-year-old diabetic could expect 1.3 years of life; a diabetic of 25 could expect 2.1 years; a diabetic of 45 could expect 8.5 years. During the Allen diet era, which lasted from 1914 until 1922, the life expectancy of the 10-year-old had doubled to 2.6 years of life; the 25-year-old's expectancy rose to four years; that of the 45-year-old climbed to 10.5 years.

Allen's Undernutrition Treatment

The Allen diet, worked out by Dr. Frederick M. Allen of the Rockefeller Institute for Medical Research, stands as America's contribution to the treatment of diabetes by systematic undernutrition. In many ways it was a development of the Guelpa semi-starvation treatment.

Under the Allen method, a patient was first fasted for several days, then put on a diet in which carbohydrates, fats, and proteins were all sharply reduced.

In a fairly typical case, treatment began with a seven-day fast during which the patient was daily allowed four bran muffins and some fluids, none of which provided any calories.

The patient was then allowed to eat for nine days, the daily calorie total rising from 64 on the first day to 504 on the ninth. There was a fast on the tenth day and, on the eleventh day, the patient was allowed 151 calories. With a fast every seven days, the calorie allowance rose until, on the thirty-fourth day of treatment, it reached 1,031 calories.

After a patient was discharged sugar-free, he had to follow a maintenance diet. This involved a fast day, most commonly every two weeks and usually on a Sunday. Dr. Allen felt that such Sundays of deprivation would help the patient in "atoning for any chance indiscretions."

Since the diet emphasized total restriction of calories, various foods were recommended which offered bulk without nutrition. One of these foods was bran, a major part of the bulk in the Allen diet. Dr. Allen suggested that coarse bran flakes commonly used for the feeding of cattle were " . . . perfectly satisfactory when washed under the cold water tap for a half an hour or more . . ."

Indigestible substitutes for flour and other carbohydrates were also suggested. One of these was talcum powder.

As a possible recipe, Dr. Allen proposed "making a batter with eggs, spices and impalpable talcum powder, and frying it crisp. This will appear more satisfying than the egg fried alone."

Dr. Allen admitted it was possible "for a few cases even under the most expert care, to end in actual death from starvation . . ." However he felt that the experience of Dr. E. P. Joslin showed that death from starvation was much less frequent than death from coma and was therefore the lesser risk.

This was the high point in the dietary treatment of diabetes when Banting and Best isolated insulin and began a medical revolution.

For the first time in history, the diabetic patient could be freed from starvation diets. Instead of having to reduce his food intake to meet his limited insulin supply, he could now inject enough insulin to allow him to eat a relatively normal diet without trouble.

That, at least, was the reality made possible by the isolation of insulin. Many doctors were slow to accept this new reality. The dogma of diet was too deeply imbedded to be easily liberalized.

Many mild diabetics can survive without insulin and with relatively minor dietary restrictions. Other patients would require diets that amount to semi-starvation. For them, survival is possible without insulin, but with insulin they could avoid extreme deprivation and live more nearly normal lives. Yet, because of the influence of the diet cult, some of these patients were denied insulin or allowed only enough to make their dietary restrictions barely tolerable. There were even many patients who would rather submit to any privations than take insulin.

For more than ten years after the introduction of insulin, treatment included a subnormal diet until increasing pressure forced gradual reform. Reluctantly, the dietary dogmas underwent modification and, along with these changes, many of the fetishes began to disappear.

Today, although they still have not vanished from the scene, there are fewer diabetics who use special scales to weigh the grams of vegetables or other foods they are permitted to eat; fewer charts on which to enter the records of grams and calories; fewer lists of permitted and forbidden foods.

In about 70 percent of the cases, practical experience has shown that the longer a person has diabetes, the more he tends to deviate from a prescribed diet until a normal food intake is approximated. As a rule, people cannot long be held to a diet that is too different from their normal eating pattern. At the Elliot P. Joslin Camp for Diabetic Boys in Charlton, Mass., 61 percent of the youngsters confessed that they did not follow a diet at home.

A study made in Sweden, where practically all diabetics are registered, bears out the resistance to diets. Only one-third of all those patients who were prescribed diets followed the instructions. The longer a patient used insulin, the more frequently he gradually changed over to a normal diet.

The Modern Diet Returns to Normal

Dietary diehards notwithstanding, it is now generally accepted that the diabetic patient's diet should approximate the nutritional allowances recommended for "normal" people by the National Research Council unless he is overweight or suffers some complication such as hyperthyroidism. In those cases there may be an increase or decrease in nutritional needs.

We also know that earlier estimates of the carbohydrate content of various foods such as string beans, broccoli, and other vegetables were too high because they include indigestible carbohydrates which could not be used by the body. These inaccuracies have been corrected by both the American Dietetic Association and the American Diabetes Association, permitting a somewhat easier diet even for those under rigid carbohydrate restriction.

The physician who treats diabetes today need no longer be a symbol of punishment and deprivation to the patient.

At least 50 percent of adult diabetics can be treated without insulin but with a diet providing a mild to moderate restriction of carbohydrates. Special diets with complicated lists of foods and permissible substitutes are not usually necessary.

Obese patients should have their weight reduced to normal. A 1,200 calorie diet usually is enough to do this. Where a weight-reducing diet weakens a patient, it might be better for him to take insulin or an oral drug and relax the diet.

For diabetics who are not obese and who show little or no sugar in the urine, the simple omission of concentrated sugars, pastry, and soft drinks is often enough. This is especially true of elderly individuals.

The average vigorous adult with mild diabetes and moderate urinary sugar might control his disease by reducing his daily carbohydrate intake and eating adequate fat and protein—meat, fish, eggs, and cheese.

A great number of mild diabetics need not bother with complicated diets at all. They can be treated by omitting from their meals sugars, syrups, pastry, and soft drinks, or by limiting carbohydrates—eating less bread, rice, potatoes or macaroni. The patient who reduces carbohydrates may increase his protein. The mild diabetic may also use alcohol in the form of cognac, rum, whiskey, or dry wines, since this can be converted to energy by a direct process that does not require insulin.

As far as possible, the diabetic's diet should be kept within the normal pattern of his eating habits. An Italian, for instance, should not be put on a corned-beef-and-cabbage diet.

Currently, a wide variety of food and soft drinks using sugar substitutes have made it possible for diabetics to enjoy sugar-free foods, drinks, and desserts previously not available to them.

Finally, a diabetic who keeps losing weight and does not have the energy he needs to work and live normally should not be treated by dietary restriction alone. He should be permitted to eat the foods that will let him feel and do his best, and be given insulin or an oral drug to help him utilize them.

Juvenile diabetics, especially children, should not have restrictive diets. Only concentrated sugars—soda pop, candy, jams, and jellies—ought to be curbed. Ice cream, cookies, even puddings usually may be eaten. Children need adequate nutrition for proper growth. They must be fed adequately and given enough insulin to help them maintain a positive metabolic balance.

Diabetics of normal weight who take insulin or Orinase do not usually have to worry about diets. They should not overeat, and they could benefit from a reduction of concentrated sugars. But they are no longer slaves to the diabetic's food scales, food lists, record charts and all the other paraphernalia that once turned the simple act of eating into a ritual involving mathematics, chemistry, bookkeeping, and self-punishment.

This does not mean that the diabetic who takes insulin may eat as he pleases. He must always be on guard to avoid the hazards of insulin shock. Here, the timing of the diet is of paramount importance. Since his daily insulin dosage is specifically geared to the timing and content of his meals, the diabetic *must* eat at the prescribed times. If he wants to avoid trouble he must be sure neither to delay nor skip a meal.

Beyond that, thanks to insulin and the oral drugs, he has been freed from the locked rooms, the starvation diets, the metabolic fasts, and the other mumbo-jumbo of the Diabetic Dark Ages. He can at last enjoy the simple pleasure of eating without the guilty feeling that he is committing a mortal metabolic sin.

CHAPTER 6

The Meaning of Insulin

If Otto Folin of Harvard had worked out his test for blood sugar in 1908 instead of 1913, insulin might have been in use 14 years earlier.

History—and medical history is no exception—is as full of bitter ironies as it is of happy accidents. Insulin, or something very much like it, was extracted from the pancreas in 1908 by a German scientist, George Zuelzer. This extract was injected into several dogs and the unfortunate animals died. Zuelzer, unable to learn exactly why the dogs died, decided that the substance was too dangerous.

A test would have shown that the insulin extract had caused so rapid a drop in blood sugar that the dogs suffered extreme insulin shock. Even without the blood sugar test, had Zuelzer used diabetic instead of healthy dogs in the tests, his extract would have produced relief of symptoms instead of shock. And Zuelzer would today be one of medicine's immortals, not an obscure scientist whose name is all but forgotten.

Still another rendezvous with immortality ended in a near miss when Israel S. Kleiner of New York and J. R. Murlin of Rochester, N.Y., produced an insulin extract. As with Zuelzer, the blood test that would have shown the importance of the work was not yet available.

Many researchers had already helped pave the way when Frederick G. Banting came upon the scene. Minkowski and von Mering had shown in 1889 that the removal of the pancreas caused a diabetes-like disease in a dog.

In 1900, Opie of Johns Hopkins had reported that in diabetics there was a degeneration in the islets of Langerhans, those mysterious small cells in the pancreas.

Then, in 1916, Sir Edward Sharpey-Schafer speculated that the islets of Langerhans produced a substance without which diabetes would develop. This was the mysterious "X" that scientists were arguing about with great heat; some feeling that it existed and was involved in diabetes; others maintaining that there was no such substance.

Allen, of Allen diet fame, was outstanding among those who opposed the possibility of "organ therapy" and felt that there was nothing in the pancreas that could be used to treat diabetes.

Piece by piece, the evidence continued to mount. There *had* to be something in the pancreas, most likely in the islets of Langerhans, that somehow had a part in the onset of diabetes.

Thus the stage was set for Frederick G. Banting of Canada. In 1920 he was a young orthopedic surgeon who found it so hard to make a living at his profession that he took up part-time teaching at the Western Ontario Medical School.

One evening, while he was preparing a lecture to be given the following day, he picked up a copy of a medical journal and was attracted by an article written by Moses Barron. What he read transformed him from a discouraged young doctor into an inspired researcher. Barron had written that when gallstones blocked the pancreatic ducts, the part of the pancreas that manufactured the digestive juices shriveled up—but the islets of Langerhans were unhurt. Furthermore, wrote Barron, when dogs had their pancreatic ducts tied off the same thing happened. The part of the pancreas that made the digestive juices degenerated, but the islet cells continued to function and the dogs lived.

Banting recalled Minkowski's work. If the whole pancreas were removed the dog died of diabetes. Now Barron seemed to supply the final clue. Where the whole pancreas was destroyed *except* the islets of Langerhans, the dogs *did not* get diabetes and die. Therefore, there had to be something in the islets of Langerhans which, if removed, produced diabetes and death.

The next step was to get at this mysterious substance. Barron had shown the way here too. By tying off the pancreatic ducts of dogs for six to eight weeks, the regular pancreatic tissue would degenerate. Then, removing what was left and making an extract of the still-functioning islets, Banting should have the answer.

The Banting-Best Breakthrough

Banting convinced Professor MacLeod of the University of Toronto Medical School that he had a promising approach to the diabetes problem. With MacLeod's backing and blessing, as well as the facilities of his laboratory, Banting went to work. As an assistant, Banting had a second-year medical student, Charles H. Best, who had, literally, tossed a coin with another student for the job.

It was a grim, heartbreaking task. Failure followed failure. Then, one day in July, 1921, just as they were teetering on the threshold of defeat, came the first glimmer of possible success. Another in a long series of extracts was made and injected into a diabetic dog—and this time the dog miraculously improved. Then it sickened again and died.

Why should the animal die? The answer seemed clear. One dose of insulin was not enough. The dog had to receive a constant supply of the mysterious substance its own missing pancreas could no longer provide.

In January, 1922, after many more setbacks, Banting and Best achieved what looked like a real experimental success. They were treating a dog—part collie and part just dog—who was diabetic and should have been dead long ago. But the dog, a female, was alive and frisky. The extract worked.

Banting and Best were ready for the really critical test—on a human being. The human guinea pig was Joe Gilchrist, one of Banting's childhood friends. Gilchrist had severe diabetes; and the Allen diet, although it kept him alive, had reduced him to a scant shadow of life.

On February 11, 1922, Joe Gilchrist became the first diabetic human being to receive an injection of insulin. He waited, waited—and then he felt a surge of new life pour through him. The rest is medical history.

Insulin—no longer a hypothetical substance whose existence doctors disputed about—had been isolated, and it worked. A way had at last been found to control the grim course of diabetes—one that would not only keep the diabetic alive but would also allow him to live.

Miraculous though it seemed at the time, the insulin extract used to treat Dr. Gilchrist was far from perfect. For one thing, it was very impure. For another, it was quite unpredictable—getting weaker and weaker in the extract for some unknown reason.

The trouble with the early insulin lay in the extraction process. Banting and Best used a mixture of alcohol and alkali to wash the insulin substance from the prepared pancreas. What they did not know, and neither did anyone else at the time, was that the alkali reacted with the insulin, gradually detroying it.

At this point, a brilliant Canadian chemist, James B. Collip, appeared on the scene to help Banting and Best improve the purity of their product. Collip not only discovered that the alkali was destroying the insulin, but that it really did a poor job extracting it from the pancreas.

Once he spotted the trouble, Collip substituted an acid for the alkali and tested it. The new alcohol-acid combination fulfilled his expectations. It extracted more insulin from the pancreas and, furthermore, had no destructive effect upon the precious substance.

Diabetics the world over heard of the discovery. Overnight, the demand for insulin went far beyond anything that could be produced from the pancreases of Banting's or any available dogs. Insulin had to be produced in vast quantities to meet the enormous need. There *had* to be some other source.

For a while, Banting and Best were able to obtain an increased amount of insulin from the pancreases of unborn calves. Since the islets of Langerhans formed first, it was not necessary to tie off the pancreatic ducts and then wait for the rest of the pancreas to degenerate. Even with this more accessible source of insulin, the demand quickly outstripped the supply.

At this critical stage, Collip's process provided a solution. His extraction technique made it possible to use the pancreases of cattle and pork *without tying off the ducts*. It also recovered a far greater amount of the available insulin.

First Steps with Insulin

All this time the experimental work went on. Insulin was good, but it had to be made better. Other scientists stepped into the picture. John Abel, a Johns Hopkins University chemist, was the first to produce pure insulin in crystalline form. This gave scientists a better opportunity to study the newly found hormone.

For diabetics, absolutely pure insulin was no boon. It did not perform at top capacity unless traces of zinc were present. So the zinc which had been purified out of the crystalline insulin was put back in.

The original insulin had no measurement of strength. Since it soon became necessary to know the concentration being used, an arbitrary measurement was arrived at and called a unit. This was the amount of insulin activity that could lower the blood sugar of a rabbit by a specific amount. This measurement unit is still in use.

When the first commercial insulin appeared it was relatively weak, providing 10 units of insulin activity per cubic centimeter. Then a more concentrated form of 20 units per cc. appeared. These weak dilutions were uneconomical to market and impractical for the patient. Today's concentrations of 40 and 80 units per cc. provide a better range for almost all patients, with one injection enough for a daily dose.

By 1927, five years after Joe Gilchrist had received his first injection, there were two standard insulins available for diabetes patients—the original regular insulin and the newer crystalline zinc insulin. Both were clear liquids which were promptly absorbed and began to act within the hour. The effect lasted three or four hours then dwindled rapidly. This created a problem.

The action was of such short duration that these insulins had to be injected before every meal and, by most patients, before going to bed. So the scientists went to work to reduce the number of daily injections.

For almost ten years all sorts of experiments were tried in the hope of finding a way to prolong the action of insulin. Various kinds of materials were combined with insulin in order to help slow it down—paraffin, tannic acid, alum. None of them worked.

Different Insulins for Different Needs

Finally, in 1935, a group of scientists under H. C. Hagedorn in Copenhagen announced that they had the answer—two answers, in fact. With this, Denmark began a virtual monopoly on insulin discoveries.

The first discovery prolonged the action of insulin so that one injection could work for 12 to 16 hours. This increase was obtained by adding to the insulin a simple protein substance called protamine, obtained from the sperm of the rainbow trout. The protamine attached itself to the insulin and caused a slower release of insulin activity. This came to be known as protamine insulin.

The second discovery was an extension of the first. Hagedorn found that by adding zinc to the protamine insulin, the action was prolonged even further and would last for more than 24 hours.

Protamine zinc insulin, a milky fluid, was made available in the United States in 1937. With the advent of the Danish-developed insulin, it became possible for most diabetics who needed moderate doses to handle their ailment with only one injection a day.

But protamine zinc insulin did not solve all the problems. There were still a number of diabetics whose insulin needs were so complicated that no one of the available insulins could give them the needed protection with a single injection.

Children, for instance, need very rapid insulin activity. Regular and crystalline zinc insulins gave them the speed they needed but did not last long enough. Protamine zinc insulin, while it gave prolonged activity, did not start soon enough.

Other diabetics whose disease was erratic found

that the protamine zinc insulin did not give enough activity during the day, when they were eating. At night, when the long-acting insulin had no food to work on, there would be too much insulin action and the patient might go into shock.

In the face of these special needs, mixed insulins came into use for juvenile, insulin-deficient diabetics. Instructed by their physicians, the patients would make the mixtures in the hypodermic syringe, combining the required quick-acting and the long-acting insulins to give them the kind of activity they needed.

These mixtures proved so useful, and their use became so widespread, that they led to the introduction by Hagedorn of Neutral Protamine Hagedorn (NPH) insulin. This insulin resembles a mixture of three parts regular and two parts protamine zinc. It is more stable than the homemade mixtures, more predictable and has greater flexibility than the unmixed insluins that preceded it. NPH has proved vitally important for children; and, for erratic diabetics, gives more activity during the day and less at night, thus easing the hazard of shock.

Two more insulins were still to come. One was globin insulin, which appeared in 1943. This consists of regular insulin to which globin, a protein from beef blood, is added to slow the action. Like regular and crystalline zinc insulins, globin insulin is a clear fluid. Unlike them, it has a long action and a slower onset of activity.

The most recent addition to the insulin family is known as Lente insulin. Developed in 1955 by Hallas-Møller of Denmark, this is made by adding sodium acetate to regular zinc insulin. The sodium acetate acts as a buffer to maintain an acid-alkali balance. Unlike the sodium phosphate buffer used in other insulins, the sodium acetate also has a slowing action of its own. This makes the addition of a protein such as globin or protamine unnecessary.

Lente—which means "slowly" in Latin—has an

action somewhere between regular and protamine zinc insulins. Its duration is about 24 hours. Although its action starts relatively fast, it is not quick enough for insulin-deficient diabetics or for emergency situations caused by acidosis and coma. In such cases, if it is used at all, it is boosted with quick-acting regular or crystalline zinc insulin.

Today's diabetic, unlike Joe Gilchrist, has a wide range of insulins at his disposal. None of these is yet the *perfect* insulin. The long-lasting one do not start soon enough, the quick-acting ones do not last long enough—and all of them have to be injected. Furthermore, while the natural insulin produced by the body is released only to the extent that it is needed at any given moment, injected insulin *cannot* synchronize its activity to the body's changing blood-sugar levels. Despite these drawbacks, the total insulin armament is complete enough to provide an answer to almost every need that may develop in diabetes.

For the diabetic, the insulin armory represents nearly total security.

In human terms, the value of insulin and what it did cannot adequately be put into words. It made life possible where there was only the certainty of death. Even more than bare life, it gave the diabetic that most precious gift of all—the opportunity to take joy in living.

There is a woman alive today who soon will be celebrating a half-century of life. Yet, had it not been for the isolation of insulin, she would most likely have been dead at 15.

She is a normal woman, happily married and vigorously anticipating the good years that still lie ahead. In 1922, she was a case history of an early insulin success.

Diabetes came upon her suddenly at the age of ten. She had been a healthy, good-natured child with a fondness for sweets when the disease struck. In two months, her weight fell from 64 pounds to 57. The year was 1918 and there was no insulin, only rigid diet. One year later, after considerable fasting, she showed some improvement and was allowed to return to school.

Not for long. Her diabetes became more severe and, aggravated by an attack of influenza, flared up. Her weight began to fall sharply and she became bedridden. By June, 1922, at the age of 14, she was a living skeleton weighing less than 47 pounds. She had to undergo 5 days of fasting to avoid passing into diabetic coma.

Three months later she was back in the hospital again to partake of a possible miracle. If the miracle worked, she might live. If it did not work . . .

The name of the miracle was insulin—and it worked.

In September she had been taking *no* insulin. Eating 470 calories a day when she was allowed anything at all, she weighed a shade under 47 pounds and, though nearing the age of 15, was inexorably withering away.

Three months later, in December, 1922, she was taking 25 units of insulin, eating 1,861 calories a day and weighed 57 pounds. Her once pathetically jutting bones steadily lost their sharpness as the flesh stopped melting away and began to form once again.

Today some 35 years later, the emaciated girl, who would have died at 15, is a wife and a matron who has completely fulfilled the promise of her womanhood.

That is the meaning of insulin.

CHAPTER 7

Control with Insulin – the Tools

All juvenile and most young adult diabetics must take insulin. All those suffering from acidosis, disability, continuing weight loss or other complications should take insulin. About half of all maturity-onset diabetics require insulin.

Altogether, about 70 percent of all diabetics need insulin. This means that of the estimated 2,000,000 diabetics in the United States, 1,400,000 must inject themselves or be injected at least once a day unless they can take Orinase—a development which we will discuss in another chapter.

Since the aim of diabetes treatment is to permit the patient to live as normally as possible, he is taught by his physician to inject himself. This allows the diabetic greater freedom. Even diabetic children can be taught to handle their own injections.

Infants, the very young, and the disabled cannot inject themselves. In those cases a parent, relative, friend, or neighbor may be required to give the injections. In some unusual circumstances, a nurse or physician may be necessary.

The diabetic who takes insulin has still another responsibility. He must test his urine for sugar, generally at least once a day depending on the nature of his diabetes. He must also be able to test his urine for acetone if the situation requires it.

These tests enable him to keep watch on his condition. If there is any change, the results should promptly be telephoned to his physician, who will then be able to judge what steps to take.

By injecting his own insulin and taking his own tests, the diabetic is free to live his life. Using the telephone as the link with his doctor, he helps make possible treatment by remote control.

Of course, the diabetic must see the doctor for periodic examinations or when there is a change in the status of the disease. Apart from that, as long as he follows the rules of his treatment, he can pretty much go his own way.

In order to be able to handle his own injections, the diabetic must have proper equipment and know how to use it. If a parent, relative, or friend must administer the injections, they, too, must know what to do.

Before we go any further into what the diabetic needs and must know to handle his injections, let us take a closer look at the different insulins and how they act:

The Insulin Armory

Regular or Crystalline Zinc Insulin: This is sometimes called plain, unmodified, or soluble insulin. It is a clear liquid and comes in round bottles containing ten cubic centimeters, the standard size for all insulin vials. It is available in two concentrations: 40 units and 80 units per cubic centimeter. These are known as U40 and U80. Crystalline zinc insulin is also available upon request in the form of U100 and U500 for patients who need huge daily doses of 200 units or more.

This insulin is quick acting, showing an effect in less than an hour. It reaches peak activity in three to four hours and activity vanishes in six to eight hours. It is the fastest acting insulin and has the shortest duration. Because of its brief action, this insulin has to be injected before each meal. It is useful in emergencies such as coma, in insulin-deficient diabetes, in unstable diabetes where sugar levels shift frequently. It is often mixed with longer-lasting insulins to give the latter a fast start.

Protamine Zinc Insulin: A cloudy liquid which *should be shaken until thoroughly mixed.* Instructions on the bottle advise against shaking; these may be disregarded, since experience has shown that proper and complete mixing is essential if the insulin dose is to be uniform. Fresh vials of this insulin should be mixed with special care because protamine zinc insulin has a tendency to clump or adhere to the glass vial after standing for any length of time.

This insulin comes in round 10-cc. vials and is sold in concentrations of U40 and U80. It is a slow-starting, long-acting insulin with onset of activity in four to eight hours, peak action in 12 to 24 hours and total length of action from 30 to 36 hours or more. Protamine zinc insulin is useful in the large majority of cases where the patient needs small to moderate doses of up to 30 or 40 units daily.

Since it has a very long period of action, patients using it may require a light snack before bedtime to avoid possible insulin shock while sleeping. The snack might consist of tea or milk and crackers.

Protamine zinc insulin is especially useful when supplemented by unmodified insulin during infections and certain special situations. It is used in mixtures in the treatment of juvenile, unstable, and severe diabetes.

Globin Zinc Insulin: This is a clear, pale amber liquid that comes in a round vial in strengths of U40 and U80. It has an intermediate action, starting to act in about two hours, reaching a peak in eight hours and disappearing in 16 to 24 hours.

Globin zinc insulin may be used by average diabetics who need less than 40 units a day. With its peak of intense activity in eight hours, this insulin is probably meant for British, European, and South American rather than United States eating habits. It is designed for those who have a hearty lunch and an afternoon tea. Therefore, the diabetic using globin zinc insulin must have an adequate noontime meal as well as a four o'clock snack of crackers and milk or tea to prevent possible insulin shock in the late afternoon.

This insulin may prove useful where a diabetic shows a sensitivity to protamine zinc insulin. It does have a disadvantage—an unpredictability of action, especially in large doses, and may wane in the early morning hours. When this happens, the diabetic is usually awakened by a need to urinate. Another disadvantage of globin zinc insulin is the fact that in about 20 percent of the patients it seems to cause a painful or burning sensation at the site of injection.

NPH (Neutral Protamine Hagedorn) Insulin: A suspension of tiny crystals which, when thoroughly mixed, becomes a cloudy fluid. It comes in square vials in U40 and U80 concentrations. In action, it resembles a mixture of three parts regular insulin with two parts protamine zinc. It provides more activity during the day and less at night; begins to act in about four hours, reaches a peak in eight hours and is used up in 24 hours.

This insulin is more flexible, stable, and easier to use than homemade mixtures. It provides insulin action that is closer to the needs of the majority of mild cases and about half the severe cases than do either protamine zinc or globin insulin. Where more rapid action is needed, as with juvenile diabetics, regular insulin may be added to NPH without loss of activity.

Because NPH crystals have an unusual tendency to settle to the bottom of the vial, especially in the cold, this type of insulin may require vigorous shaking to make sure it is evenly mixed. If any crystals are visible, shake thoroughly, even if foaming does result in the vial.

Lente Insulin: This is a combination of two other insulins: 30 percent Semilente and 70 percent Ultralente insulins. *Semilente* is a suspension of regular insulin, has a rapid action within one to two hours and endures up to 12 hours. *Ultralente* is a suspension of zinc-insulin crystals, has a very slow starting action and a duration of 36 hours or more. Lente, combining these two insulins, comes in hexagonal vials in concentrations of U40 and U80. It has a fairly rapid onset of action, about one or two hours, and a duration of 32 hours or more.

It may meet the needs of most average diabetics with a single injection a day as do NPH, globin, or protamine zinc insulins; and often it also needs a boost of regular insulin for juvenile and severe diabetics. Like globin insulin, Lente has been found by some diabetics to cause a painful or burning sensation at the site of the injection.

For a number of cases where Lente is not suitable, Ultralente and Semilente are now available to provide tailor-made mixtures to fit the patient's special need.

These are the various insulins. Alone or in varying combinations, they are used to manage those cases of diabetes which cannot comfortably be controlled by other means.

The accompanying insulin chart should prove useful for ready reference:

INSULIN CHART

Type of Insulin	Appear- ance	Vial Shape	Action begins in	Action lasts
Regular	Clear	Round	1 hour	4 hrs.
Crystalline Zinc	Clear	Round	1 hour	4 hrs.
Protamine Zinc	Cloudy	Round	4 to 6 hrs.	24 to 32 hrs.
NPH	Cloudy	Square	4 hrs.	24 hrs.
Lente	Cloudy	Hexagonal	1 to 2 hrs.	24 to 32 hrs.
Globin Zinc	Clear	Round	4 hrs.	18 to 24 hrs.
Semilente	Cloudy	Hexagonal	1 to 2 hrs.	To 12 hrs.
Ultralente	Cloudy	Hexagonal	6 to 8 hrs.	36 hrs.

The kind of insulin a diabetic takes depends upon the nature of his ailment and is determined by his physician. The diabetic's doctor will tell him what kind of insulin to use, the size of the dose, when and how to inject it, what precautions to take against the possibilities of diabetic acidosis and insulin shock.

Things to Know About Insulin

Very few diabetics have a true allergy to insulin. But during the early weeks of treatment, 10 to 20 percent of the patients using insulin have minor reactions consisting of local itching, swelling or pain. Ordinarily these symptoms vanish by themselves after two or three weeks. If they persist or are more severe, the doctor may prescribe oral antihistamines or he may, in some cases, recommend that an antihistamine be mixed in the syringe with the insulin.

In some cases the diabetic may have an allergy to beef or pork protein. In that event insulin from mixed sources should be avoided. As soon as the nature of the allergy is determined, a special insulin derived from the non-allergy-producing source can be obtained from Eli Lilly and Co., which produces separate insulins from beef pancreas and pork pancreas as well as from mixed sources.

Many diabetics often want to know which company makes which insulins.

Eli Lilly & Co. makes all forms of insulin.

E. R. Squibb and Sons makes all forms but Lente. Merck Sharp & Dohme makes all but Lente and globin insulins.

Burroughs Wellcome & Co. makes only globin insulin.

Here are some other facts about insulin which diabetics should know:

Each vial of insulin has an expiration date. Ordinarily, the insulin will remain active beyond that date but, except in emergencies where no fresh insulin is available, outdated insulin should not be used. *Unopened vials of outdated insulin can be returned to the pharmacist and exchanged, without cost, for a fresh vial.*

Most diabetics will also find that they can save considerable money over a period of years by buying vials of U80 rather than U40 insulin. Since packaging enters into the cost of insulin, one U80 vial of 800 units will cost less than two U40 vials of 400 units each. In a lifetime disease such as diabetes, the saving can be substantial.

There are still other factors in favor of using U80 insulin wherever possible.

The higher concentration of the U80 insulin requires a smaller volume of injected insulin. A U80 injection of 40 units requires only ½ cc. as against a full 1 cc. if U40 insulin is used. The smaller volume is less likely to cause local skin reactions and other disturbances.

The severe diabetic's average insulin dose is about 70 units. This can be taken in the standard 1-cc. syringe only by using U80 insulin.

The U40 concentration is important where the prescribed dose is less than 10 units. In these cases the higher U80 concentration would be hard to measure accurately.

One more fact about insulin before we turn to the equipment needed by the diabetic. *Insulin need not be refrigerated.* Refrigeration is required by law when insulin is stored or kept by the pharmacist. Despite this, insulin that is being used keeps perfectly well at average room temperature.

Protamine zinc and globin insulins are more sensitive to temperature changes than other insulins. But even these may be kept at room temperature for the period they are being used. Only the reserve supply need be stored in a cool place. *Furthermore, too much cold as well as too much heat can spoil insulin.* This is important to diabetics who have to travel, as we will show in the following chapter.

The Insulin Equipment

The diabetic who uses insulin *must* have certain equipment available at all times:

1. INSULIN

The type prescribed by his physician in the proper concentration. An extra vial or two should be kept in reserve in a cool place. Every diabetic should also have a vial of regular insulin on hand in the event of some emergency such as acidosis or coma.

2. SYRINGE

The standard insulin syringe approved by the American Diabetes Association and manufactured by Becton, Dickinson and Co. of New Jersey is preferable. One-cc. models are available for either U40 or U80 concentrations of insulin. The U40 model has the unit graduations marked in red; the U80 model is marked in green. The colors match the stoppers of the corresponding insulin vials. All U40 vials have red circles on the stoppers. Stoppers of the U80 vials have green circles. A similar syringe is the Vim, manufactured by the MacGregor Instrument Company. The syringe used should be matched to the strength of the insulin, since this will prevent errors in dosage. Diabetics who require 80 to 160 units of insulin daily will find that the 2-cc. standard U80 syringe is very useful. There are even special syringes for blind diabetics. In all cases, an extra syringe should be kept on hand against the possibility of loss or breakage.

3. HYPODERMIC NEEDLE

The needle should be of rustless or stainless steel, $1/2$ to $5/8$ inches long. It should be 25-to 26-gauge. A finer gauge, such as 27, may be used *only* with regular and globin insulin. The other insulins would tend to clog. Twenty-five- to 26-gauge needles, however, can be used with any insulin. As for the type of point, an ordinary beveled point retains its sharpness better than the more expensive Huber point. A reserve supply of needles should always be kept on hand because needles may bend or break and, in any case, usually become dull after about two weeks' use.

4. A STERILE CASE FOR SYRINGE AND NEEDLE

This is convenient for home use and is essential for travel. Elaborate outfits are available, but the simplest is probably the B-D Steritube No. 300 (No. 350 for larger syringes) or the Vim case. These can be sterilized by boiling along with the syringe and needle. Filled with alcohol, the interiors will remain sterile for one to two weeks and will keep the syringe and needle sterile for that time.

5. ALCOHOL AND STERILE COTTON

These are essential for sterilization of the top of the insulin vial which will be punctured by the needle and for the site of the injection. Pure grain ethyl alcohol is *not* essential. Denatured and isopropyl alcohol—ordinary rubbing alcohol—does the job just as well *and is much less expensive*.

6. AMPULES OF GLUCAGON

These should be on hand in the event of insulin

shock and similar emergencies. Glucagon will raise the blood sugar when it is too low or when too much insulin has been taken. Like insulin, this hormone can be injected by any member of the family in the event the patient cannot do it for himself and is unable to take sweets by mouth to counteract shock.

It is prepared by Eli Lilly and Co. and comes in a vial as a powder which is diluted by liquid in an accompanying vial. The entire amount of the diluted powder is injected.

7. TESTS FOR URINARY SUGAR

Clinitest, Clinistix, or Tes-Tape are available. Since daily urine tests are needed in a great many cases, one of these is essential equipment. Clinistix only shows the presence or absence of sugar. The others also show the amount of sugar.

8. TESTS FOR URINARY ACETONE

The majority of mild diabetics probably will not need this but, in any case, three fairly simple tests are available—Ketostix, Acetest, and Acetone Test Powder. One of these should be kept on hand for emergencies and in those more extreme cases where acetone tests are important.

9. AN IDENTIFICATION CARD

Every diabetic who takes insulin should carry a card with his name, address, and phone number as well as those of his physician. The card should also state that he is diabetic and should carry the following request:

"If I am unconscious or behaving abnormally I may be having an insulin reaction.

"If I can swallow, give me sugar, candy, fruit juice or a sweetened drink. If I cannot swallow or do not recover promptly, call a physician or send me to the hospital at once."

Standard cards may be obtained free from any affiliates of the American Diabetes Association; Eli Lilly & Co., 740 S. Alabama St., Indianapolis 6, Ind.; The Upjohn Company, Kalamazoo, Mich.; the U.S. Vitamin & Pharmaceutical Corp., 800 Second Ave., New York 17, N.Y.; or from E. R. Squibb and Sons, 745 Fifth Avenue, New York 22, N.Y.

These nine pieces of equipment are necessary for the diabetic who takes insulin. They should provide him with all he needs to manage the disease. Many other things are made and sold but, except in special cases, are usually unnecessary and merely succeed in adding expense and clutter to the diabetic's life.

There are, for instance, several automatic injectors for diabetics who are reluctant to push a needle into themselves. This should be avoided unless absolutely necessary because it adds an unnecessary gadget and may contaminate the needle.

With this equipment, the diabetic who needs insulin should be adequately armed to deal with his disease.

CHAPTER 8

Control with Insulin – the Techniques

There is nothing very complicated about an insulin injection. A patient usually learns how to administer it from the physician or nurse. Furthermore, the whole process is shown pictorially in various pamphlets which can be obtained free of charge from the American Diabetes Association, Eli Lilly & Co., The Upjohn Co., Chas. Pfizer & Co., U.S. Vitamin & Pharmaceutical Corp., or from E. R. Squibb and Sons.

Still, the procedure is so important that it is worth reviewing:

1. The syringe and needle must be sterilized by boiling in water for about five minutes or by constant immersion in alcohol in a "Steritube" or similar case. In the event such a case is used, then it, the syringe and needle should be sterilized by boiling *at least* once every two weeks. Since hard water tends to cake the syringe and needle, make sure soft water is used. If necessary, use distilled water or a commercial water softener. Hard water can usually be detected by a whitish residue it leaves as it boils away.

2. Make sure the insulin to be used is completely mixed in the vial. Only globin, regular, and crystalline-zinc insulins need no mixing. If a mixture of insulins is made in the syringe, make sure they are *thoroughly* mixed.

3. Be careful to eject any water or alcohol from the syringe.

4. Wash the site of the injection with soap and water, then apply alcohol with a cotton dab. Injections should be made in the arms, legs, or abdomen, and *a different site in a different area should be used each time.*

5. Wipe the rubber stopper in the insulin vial with another piece of cotton wet with alcohol. *Never remove the stopper.*

6. Set the plunger of your syringe at the mark showing your dose.

7. Stick the needle through the rubber stopper of the vial and push the plunger all the way in. This forces air into the vial.

8. Turn the vial slowly upside down several times, then with the vial upside down, pull the plunger back to the mark showing your dose. If there are any air bubbles in the syringe, push the plunger in slowly then pull it back to your proper dosage mark once more. *Be absolutely sure your proper*

dose is in the syringe before you withdraw the needle from the vial.

9. Contrary to most instructions, there is no need to pinch the skin. Hold it steady and stick the needle into the site of the injection quickly and deeply *with the needle going straight in,* not at an angle. Push the plunger in *slowly* as far as it will go.

10. Hold the piece of cotton wet with alcohol lightly over the spot where the needle enters the skin. Then pull out the needle, continuing to hold the cotton on the skin for a few seconds. *Do not rub the injection site.* Just press.

11. Take the syringe apart and rinse with clear water or, if a Steritube or Vim case is being used, return it to the tube.

These are the steps in taking an insulin injection. It is important to observe them carefully to avoid contaminating the insulin, as well as the danger of injecting too much or not enough insulin. The process is not at all complicated once it is practiced a few times. Child diabetics, no more than four years of age, have been taught to give themselves their own injections.

Insulin Demands Rigid Eating Schedule

Since various insulins have differing times of action, the diabetic must be careful to adjust his meal schedule to the timing of his injections. A change in type of insulin may require a change in eating time.

Injections should also be made the same time each day. If an injection of long-acting insulin is delayed several hours one day, the extended action into the following day may cause too rapid a drop in blood sugar if the next injection is taken on time.

On the other hand, if there is going to be an expected delay in breakfast due, say, to the partaking of Holy Communion, there should be a 25 percent reduction in the dose of long-acting insulin the day before.

There is one fact a diabetic should keep constantly in mind. If he takes insulin it is absolutely essential for him to keep to a rigidly fixed schedule of eating. Even if he has no other dietary restrictions whatsoever, *he must eat at the proper times imposed by the action of the insulin he takes.*

Meals may not be skipped or delayed. They may not be consolidated.

Certain types of insulin even require that the diabetic take between-meal snacks. NPH and globin insulins, since they reach a high peak of action in the late afternoon, make a snack *imperative* at 4 P.M. This may be a sandwich or crackers and milk or tea. These insulins also make bedtime snacks permissible, but not necessary.

Protamine zinc insulin, on the other hand, if taken in moderate or large doses *demands* a snack before bedtime and makes permissible a crackers-and-milk snack in the late afternoon.

The absolute need for balance between meals, mealtimes and insulin injections should not be hard to understand.

In order to function normally, every human being needs a certain level of sugar in the blood. If this level of sugar rises too high, we have the symptoms of diabetes; if it falls too low, our nervous systems and brains cannot function normally and we may even develop symptoms of acidosis.

When a diabetic injects insulin, he must be sure that there will always be just enough carbohydrate in his system for the insulin to act upon without upsetting the normal balance. If he eats too much or too frequently for his insulin dose, excess sugar will accumulate in his system. If he eats too little, misses a meal or eats irregularly, at some time during the day the insulin he has injected will have no free carbohydrate to work on. It will therefore go to work on the normally-needed sugar in the blood, nerve and brain tissue, burning it up and causing a sugar shortage—

a condition known as hypoglycemia which, unless it is promptly corrected, results in insulin shock.

Insulin and Physical Activity

In addition to making sure his meals and mealtimes are matched to the action of his insulin injections, the diabetic must also try to keep his physical activity as regular as possible. If he is abnormally active, over-exerts himself or misses too much sleep, more than the usual amount of sugar is used up, thus leaving less for the insulin to act upon.

Where the variable physical activity is predictable, the insulin dose can be adjusted in advance. A laborer needs less insulin during the week when his work is burning up much sugar than he does on weekends when his major activity is watching television.

In many cases, modern civilization makes it difficult to know in advance when we will be required to pro-duce a burst of physical activity. A man may have to run to catch a train; a woman may have to do emer-gency cleaning and shopping because of the arrival of unexpected guests; a child may get into a fight or a game and suddenly overexert himself.

Wherever possible, the diabetic must learn how to meet these emergencies. Where he cannot adjust the insulin dosage, he might find it advisable—when physi-cal overactivity is unavoidable—to protect himself with some rapidly available carbohydrate such as candy, a "coke," fruit or fruit juice.

Under most circumstances, the average diabetic who is alert to changing situations and intelligent about his ailment is able to meet emergencies with little if any trouble.

As a matter of fact, it is absolutely astounding that so many patients can be entrusted with self-adminis-tration of so potent a drug as insulin and, despite human error and the daily vicissitudes of life, do so effective a job. It is an utterly unique phenomenon unmatched by anything else in medicine.

With the emphasis on making life as normal as possible, there is no reason why the average diabetic should have any qualms about traveling or taking a vacation—going off on a hunting or fishing trip.

Naturally, he must watch his eating schedule and energy output and keep them in balance with his insulin dosage.

He must take all his necessary equipment with him and have spares of everything available.

He need *not* buy expensive, insulated kits in which to carry his insulin. He *must* be sure that he neither freezes nor overheats his insulin; and that everything he needs for his injections is readily at hand—not packed away in some luggage compartment.

If he is using a plane, insulin placed with the baggage in an unheated baggage compartment will freeze; therefore, he should carry it on his person. If he is traveling by car, insulin kept in the glove compartment may overheat in the summer. So the diabetic must be sure he carries his insulin in such a way that extremes of heat and cold are avoided.

As for sterilizing his syringe, if he uses a Steritube or Vim case, he can sterilize the syringe, needle, and tube before he leaves on his vacation and, by observing the normal precautions when he uses his syringe, not have to sterilize it again for as long as two weeks.

New sterile, disposable plastic syringes with needles are available to be used once and discarded. These are increasingly popular for travel. Wrapped in sterile paper, they cost ten to fifteen cents each, and the price is declining as production increases.

Testing for Sugar and Acetone

Now we come to another task the insulin-taking diabetic must perform if he is to enjoy the freedom that comes with self-treatment. He must test his urine for sugar and, under certain circumstances, for acetone which appears when fat is used by the body in place of sugar.

The need for testing depends on the nature of the diabetes. The mild diabetic who does not require insulin need not test his urine except during illness or if he is not feeling up to scratch.

If, under these circumstances, sugar does show up, he should test three times daily for two days. If the sugar persists, he should notify his doctor. The mild diabetes may have become aggravated and a change in treatments may be necessary.

The average adult diabetic taking insulin should test his urine for sugar each morning before breakfast. This is a guide to the adequacy of the insulin dose. If sugar is present, an increase in insulin may be necessary. If the insulin dose remains stable, the diabetic might be able to test for sugar every other day with safety. And he need not test for acetone.

If he starts to lose weight he should test twice daily, before breakfast and before dinner. If there is a sharp rise in sugar before breakfast and before the evening meal, he should also test for acetone and inform his physician by telephone. An increase in insulin may be indicated.

If he feels nausea and vomits, the diabetic should test for both sugar and acetone because either an insulin or carbohydrate shortage may be the cause—and the doctor *must* know which it is.

The juvenile diabetic should test for sugar twice daily, before breakfast and before the evening meal. If the sugar test is markedly positive for two tests, there should be a test for acetone.

During any illness, even if it is a common cold, and whether the patient is adult or juvenile, there should be at least three tests a day to check the adequacy of the insulin dose.

In any case, whether the patient is adult or juvenile, or whatever the nature of the diabetes, if the tests show any change from the normal situation the physician should be telephoned.

It is this self-testing, together with the telephone,

that makes treatment by remote control possible and gives the diabetic a far greater amount of freedom than would otherwise be possible.

Of the sugar tests available today, the simplest are *Clinitest* and *Clinistix,* marketed by the Ames Co. Inc., and *Tes-Tape,* put out by Eli Lilly & Co. Of these, *Clinitest* is probably the most accurate in showing the precise amounts of sugar in the urine; *Clinistix* and *Tes-Tape* are undoubtedly the most convenient.

Clinitest is a modern simplification of the Benedict test which was the test of choice until recently. The ingredients formerly in Benedict Solution are now combined in a tablet with sodium hydroxide to provide heating action which, in the Benedict test, required boiling water. Five drops of urine are measured into a test tube which comes with the test kit. To this, ten drops of water are added. Then a Clinitest tablet is dropped into the tube. As it dissolves it gives off heat and causes bubbling. When the bubbling stops the liquid has changed color. If it is blue, no sugar is present. If it is green, the amount of sugar is slight, ½ percent. If it is yellow, about 1 percent sugar is present. Orange indicates more than 1 percent. Orange-red shows more than 2 percent.

Clinistix are impregnated strips of paper that look like oversized matches. The test end of Clinistix should be dipped into urine or moistened by a drop of urine. If the moistened end turns blue in about a minute, sugar is present (*opposite reaction to Clinitest*). If no blue color develops, the urine is sugar-free.

Tes-Tape is a roll of yellow paper which comes in a container similar to Scotch tape. It is impregnated with a dye and the enzyme glucose oxidase which, in the presence of sugar, reacts and liberates the dye. To use it, tear off about 1½ inches of tape, dip it into a urine specimen and hold it for about a minute. Then compare it with the color chart that comes with the package. If the color of the tape remains yellow, there is no sugar. If it turns blue, about 2 percent sugar is present. *It should be noted that the color reactions are opposite to those of Clinitest.*

The modern tests for acetone in the urine are equally simple. The Ames Company puts out *Ketostix,* an impregnated paper strip, and *Acetest,* which uses a tablet; the Denver Chemical Company has *Acetone Test Powder.*

Put a drop of urine on either the Acetest tablet or on a pinch of Acetone Test Powder or dip a Ketostix strip into the urine. If the color does not change, no acetone is present. If it turns lavender, some acetone is present. If it turns deep purple, a large amount of acetone is present.

With these basic tests—and with the equipment to give himself injections—the insulin-taking diabetic is able to handle his ailment more or less by himself and with the minimum of dependence on doctor or hospital visits.

Emergencies do arise occasionally, making the physical presence of a doctor necessary at times other than those of the regular check-up examinations.

Apart from illness, infection, or some change in the course of the diabetes itself, there are the questions of insulin shock and diabetic coma which will be discussed in a later chapter. There is also the complication known as fat atrophy.

Fat atrophy due to insulin is found in about 20 percent of all patients. Normally, we all have a layer of fat under the skin. Where atrophy occurs, this fat disappears in the area where insulin is injected, leaving deep hollows. This may happen at only one injection site; it may happen at all sites.

Children and adult females are most susceptible to this complication. It is rare among men. Among children, it may clear up as they get older. Among adults, fat atrophy seems irreversible.

The cause of this condition is unknown and there is no known cure. However, it may help to avoid sensitive sites, to keep changing them and to use smaller amounts of more highly concentrated insulin.

Apart from these dangers, the average diabetic who takes insulin can—within the framework of his treatment—live a virtually normal life. He can work, play, marry, become a parent and do just about anything else that a non-diabetic can do. In short, insulin has made it possible for even the severe diabetic to live with his disease.

With the advent of Orinase and similar oral drugs, still another revolution is taking place in the treatment of diabetes. Already many diabetics who needed insulin have been freed from the need for daily injections, rigid mealtime schedules and from the ever-present possibility of shock. With these oral drugs, we stand at the opening of a new era in the control of diabetes.

CHAPTER 9

Orinase and the Oral Drugs

While the epoch-making discovery of insulin provided the diabetic with a means of controlling his disease, it also created a whole new set of problems.

To some, injections are painful and unpleasant. To others they are a distinct hardship. Still others find it impossible to inject themselves and must have it done for them—usually by a member of the family or by a friend trained to do the job.

What is more, the insulin-sensitive diabetic faces the hazards of insulin shock, and even those who are not sensitive must observe a rigid schedule of eating and physical activity.

Almost from the moment insulin was put into use, diabetics and their physicians began to hope for some safe, effective, and inexpensive treatment that could do what insulin did but that need not be injected.

Insulin pills or capsules were out of the question. Almost since its isolation researchers have been trying to find some way insulin could be administered orally. So far, the problem has been insoluble. The reason: Insulin is a protein substance which cannot be swallowed and absorbed into the system without being destroyed by the digestive juices.

So, while a few scientists continued to look for some way to make an insulin that could be taken by mouth, others, turned their attention to other possible substances. The problem was to find something which could be taken by mouth to reduce high blood sugar, help the body metabolize carbohydrates and—at the same time—produce no dangerous reactions. This last requirement proved one of the major obstacles. Drugs were found that could reduce blood sugar, but they also damaged the kidneys, liver or other organs.

Remedies were hunted almost everywhere. Some investigators tried herbs such as mushrooms, carrots, and whortleberry leaves. Some used onion juice, yeast extracts, and microbes from the intestines of birds. Not even the lore of witch doctors was overlooked as "cures" were tried from the jungles of Africa and North Borneo.

In 1926, a group of German scientists headed by Dr. E. Frank announced that they had developed an effective chemical which could be taken by mouth to reduce blood sugar. This was a relative of a substance found in turnip juice and earthworms; and it was named Synthalin.

Synthalin was brought to the market much too rapidly and, while it appears to have been effective in lowering blood sugar, it also produced serious damage to the liver in more than 40 percent of the patients who used it. The drug was therefore discontinued.

Accident Provides Clue to Oral Drug

The first hint in the 30-year search which ultimately led to Orinase came as the result of a medical accident. A group of French chemists had produced a sulfa drug variation which they thought might be taken by mouth to treat typhoid. In the early part of 1942, they sent it to the Montpellier Clinic for Contagious Diseases in Southern France where Marcel Janbon began to test it on typhoid patients.

Shortly after the drug was administered, some of the patients developed unusual symptoms. They began to perspire, became faint and dizzy; they trembled and became disoriented. Two of the patients, a girl of 19 and a woman of 31, died.

Puzzled by these effects, Janbon consulted a brilliant young physiologist at the University of Montpellier, Dr. Auguste Loubatières. Immediately suspecting that the anti-typhoid drug had produced symptoms resembling insulin shock, Loubatières began a series of tests on laboratory animals.

He found that his suspicion had been correct. The sulfa drug, known as 2254-RP, did lower blood sugar. However, it only did this when some part of the pancreas was present and, apparently, some insulin was being produced in the body. Where there were no insulin-producing islets of Langerhans, 2254-RP was ineffective.

Since this particular sulfa drug was not safe for use in humans, Loubatières went to work with a number of related drugs and published a series of papers on the results of his efforts. For some reason, perhaps because of the war and the fact that France had been overwhelmed by the Germans, this path-breaking work by Loubatières was generally overlooked. Scientists, even in the United States, knew about it—yet, incredibly, it was ignored.

Despite this, Loubatières stubbornly continued his

work, studying the manner in which various sulfa drugs acted to reduce blood sugar in the body. It was not until Orinase became generally accepted that his vital contributions received belated recognition.

The second step along the path to an oral anti-diabetes drug was almost an exact duplication of the first. This time, the scene was Berlin, and the time was 1954—twelve years after the tests at Montpellier.

Karl Joachim Fuchs, a young resident at the Augusta-Viktoria Hospital in Berlin, received a newly developed sulfa drug from his superior, Hans Franke, and was asked to test its germ-killing possibilities.

It was a fairly routine assignment since many new drugs were constantly being tested. So Fuchs administered it to patients suffering from various infections such as pneumonia and other ailments. This new drug was named BZ-55.

Apparently BZ-55 was an effective germ killer. Many patients showed prompt relief following administration of the drug. But, here and there, Fuchs noted peculiar reactions. Some patients were perspiring violently, shaking, dizzy, and confused. They reacted exactly as though they were approaching a state similar to insulin shock.

So Fuchs decided to try BZ-55 on himself. He swallowed several tablets and watched the developing symptoms of perspiration, faintness, dizziness, trembling, and hunger. A test of his blood sugar showed it had dropped far below normal.

When the results were reported to Franke, an expanded series of tests were begun. Diabetic patients were taken off insulin and given BZ-55 in its place. The drug showed itself effective in about 80 percent of the cases. It brought blood-sugar down to normal and seemed to provide generally good control.

Concurrently, in Hamburg, Germany, Ferdinand Bertram was trying BZ-55 on a group of diabetic patients at the Barmbek General Hospital. The results were startlingly like those in Berlin.

Juvenile and insulin-deficient diabetics were *not*

helped by the drug. But adult-onset diabetics showed amazingly good results.

Reports of the new drug were received with considerable caution in the United States. This was due to a number of factors, among which was the unhappy fact that Synthalin had proved toxic.

Eli Lilly & Co. of Indianapolis brought BZ-55 to the United States and gave it out for testing. In October, 1956, after considerable investigation and trial on human volunteers, the drug was withdrawn. It *was* highly effective, American researchers agreed, but in about five percent of the cases it was said to produce dangerous side reactions. In this respect, American findings disagreed with those in Germany and other European countries where the drug was announced as safe and was put into regular use.

Sugar Control with Minimal Side Effects

BZ-55 is a germ-killing sulfa drug and these drugs are known to have side reactions associated with their anti-bacterial activity. This brought a focus of interest on a sulfa-related drug which had *no* germ-killing qualities but *did* reduce blood sugar.

This new drug was developed in Germany in 1954 at the laboratories of the Farbwerke Hoechst Company. Called *tolbutamide*, this chemical is a sulfonyl-urea, related to the sulfas but not a true sulfa itself. It has absolutely no effect upon bacteria and apparently produces none of the side reactions usually connected with its germ-killing cousins.

Doctors in various parts of Germany tested it on more than 780 diabetics in a series of preliminary trials and reported that it was effective in more than half of the cases, producing remarkably slight side reactions.

The possibilities looked so promising that The Upjohn Co. of Kalamazoo, Michigan, brought the drug into the United States and, showing extreme caution, subjected the drug to one of the most careful investigations undergone by any substance in modern medical history.

The drug, known as Rastinon abroad, was given the trade name of Orinase in the United States and Canada. It was received by Upjohn in November, 1955, and put to preliminary laboratory tests on various animals including dogs, rabbits, chickens, ducks, and frogs. C. J. O'Donovan of Upjohn, who was responsible for evaluating the results of the tests, was interested in first obtaining some standard of reference as to the drug's safety, efficiency, and proper dosage levels.

After these factors were established, a number of outstanding specialists in the field of diabetes were asked to begin preliminary tests on human patients in carefully controlled hospital environments where each reaction could be accurately checked. After about two months of this testing, sufficient data had been collected to permit the start of large-scale tests which began in February, 1956.

What O'Donovan and the others involved in the testing wanted to know was the following:

Was Orinase safe?

Was there any toxicity and, if so, to what degree?

How effective was it; to what degree and in which areas?

What was the mode of action—how did it work?

In order to obtain this information, Orinase was given out to a large number of qualified physicians for tests on non-hospitalized patients on the widest possible scale. The purpose here was to obtain the broadest case experience, including tests with all sorts of diabetics, in order to learn the exact area and degree of the drug's usefulness.

It was essential to establish whether Orinase, in addition to being safe, would work in adult-onset diabetes; juvenile diabetes; whether it would be useful where the diabetes was complicated by other factors such as Addison's Disease, for instance.

By the time Orinase was finally released to physicians for general use by the Food and Drug Administration in June, 1957, it had been tested on about 20,000 selected patients. More than 3,000 physicians were involved in these tests, and detailed reports on 7,000 cases were received from 400 physicians and clinics.

These reports were evaluated individually by O'Donovan for comments by physicians and other data which could not be handled on a mass statistical level. Then the reports were turned over to a staff which processed them through IBM calculators for statistical analysis and evaluation—a job that would have been virtually impossible for humans.

The results showed that a safe and effective oral drug had at last been found.

Orinase was *not* an insulin substitute. It was not effective in *every* case where insulin was being used. But, for about half of the diabetics who took insulin, Orinase offered better diabetes control than insulin.

The largest group of tests was conducted by physicians associated with New York City's Mount Sinai Hospital where Orinase was tested on about 700 diabetics who were private, ambulatory patients. The results were typical of those in the rest of the country.

Where the patients were over 40, Orinase was effective in four out of five cases.

Where the patients were between 20 and 40, Orinase helped one out of three cases.

In juvenile diabetes and where the patients were under 20, Orinase was rarely effective.

Not a single serious or significant toxic effect was demonstrated in the entire group over a one-year period.

Upjohn's collected data, as analyzed by the IBM calculators, added to this by showing that there is no relation between the length of time a person has had diabetes and his response to Orinase. Long-standing cases showed good response as did new cases. Nor was body type of the patient a factor in response to Orinase.

Finally, in the vast nationwide test only one percent of the patients showed side effects. These were generally mild rashes which vanished even though the drug was continued. *None of the side effects were serious.*

Clearly, for a large number of diabetics, Orinase presaged a revolution in treatment virtually as great as that brought about by the discovery of insulin.

Oral Drugs—Their Mode of Action

The success of Orinase led to various modifications of the basic formula in an effort to find more effective forms. Several that were developed failed because of toxicity. Three modifications, however, were put into general use several years after Orinase.

One of these is Diabinese, known chemically as chlorpropamide, manufactured by Chas. Pfizer & Co. This is a chlorinated form of the basic sulfonylurea structure. It has increased potency—five to six times greater than that of Orinase.

Unfortunately, along with greater potency, it has a higher incidence of toxicity and side effects, particularly in the first weeks of administration. Its advantage lies in the fact that a smaller dose is required—never more than two pills daily, and its prolonged action makes a single administration a day possible.

In 1964, Eli Lilly & Co. introduced Dymelor, chemically called acetohexamide, another form of the basic sulfonylurea. Its potency is intermediate between Orinase and Diabinese.

Tolinase chemically called Tolazimide, was introduced by Upjohn in 1966, and is more potent than Orinase or Dymelor. All these sulfonylureas act by stimulating an increased release of insulin from the pancreas.

An entirely different oral drug has also been developed by the U.S. Vitamin & Pharmaceutical Corp. This is known as DBI, or phenformin.

Unlike the sulfonylureas, the action of DBI does not duplicate the effect of insulin but lowers the blood sugar in some manner not yet understood.

Certainly the immediate impact of oral therapy on the treatment of diabetes was extraordinary. In June, 1957, when Orinase was first released by the Food and Drug Administration, about 20,000 patients had used it in carefully controlled tests. By 1964, 1,250,000 diabetics in the United States were taking oral drugs.

Like insulin, the oral drugs are not the perfect answer to diabetes. They are *not* a cure. They are only a form of treatment. They are easier to use than insulin, offer fewer complications, and permit greater freedom of living habits. But, where they can replace insulin therapy in *many* cases, they cannot replace insulin in *all* cases.

For the oral drugs to work, some part of the pancreas must be present and in working order. In no case have they been known to work where the pancreas has been removed or where the islets of Langerhans were destroyed.

Nor are oral drugs indicated in severe diabetes, in juvenile or insulin-deficient diabetes, or in cases where the diabetic is severely ill, undergoing surgery, or suffering acidosis. But, even in these situations, there appear to be some areas where they *do* work. Which further emphasizes that diabetes is a disease—or group of diseases—where a vast amount of exploration remains to be done, and where the exceptions frequently *upset* the rules.

For example, oral drugs are generally not effective in juvenile diabetes according to the results of much valid testing. Yet, a small number of juvenile diabetics have responded favorably to Orinase. Physicians simply run routine tests to see how patients respond to the new drug and whether they can be changed over. Occasionally, patients who, according to statistics, *cannot* be changed over, make the change with no difficulty. In other cases, patients who should have no trouble at all cannot be changed.

Why or how this should be so is one of the mysteries of diabetes that remains to be explained.

Ordinarily, oral drugs can best replace insulin where the need for insulin is about 40 units or less daily. In some exceptional cases, patients receiving 60 or even 100 units of insulin daily have successfully changed to oral therapy. Yet . . .

A woman of 38, diabetic and unmarried, was so resistant to insulin that not even 100 units daily could control her disease. The dosage was increased, but she became progressively weaker. According to the rules, Orinase could not possibly help her. Her physician, nevertheless, decided to see if she could be changed over anyway. If she could not, nothing would be lost by trying. The change proved successful. Orinase worked and the control of this woman's diabetes is far better than it had been with insulin.

Treating the Diabetic with Oral Drugs

Oral drugs either work well or they do not work at all. This fact makes it simple for the physician to determine whether oral therapy is practicable.

Such a decision has to be made whenever a patient is newly diagnosed as diabetic. It may also become necessary with the established diabetic, one who has previously been treated with diet alone or with insulin injections and diet.

Where the patient who is being treated with dietary restriction alone shows failing results in control of the disease, he becomes a likely candidate for oral therapy.

Similarly, the established diabetic who has not been treated at all should be considered for oral treatment.

As for the insulin-treated patient, there are a number of reasons that might make him suitable for one of the oral drugs. The patient might be unwilling or unable to take the injections. He might develop an insulin allergy. For these or other reasons, the physician might decide his patient a proper subject for one of the pills.

Where this is the case, probably the easiest way to effect a change to oral therapy is by a gradual withdrawal of insulin. Parallel with this withdrawal, maximum doses of the oral drug—if it is a sulfonylurea—are administered until the insulin is completely discontinued. If the diabetes remains under control, the dose of sulfonylurea is then gradually reduced to the smallest dose required to maintain this control. However, if there is any sign that the disease is not being controlled, the patient should be returned to insulin at once.

In contrast, patients who have not taken insulin in the past—whether these are newly diagnosed diabetics or individuals who have been treated with diet or received no treatment at all—are given initially small doses of any oral drug. These are then gradually increased until control is achieved.

The maximum maintenance daily dose for the sulfonylurea drugs would be, generally, six tablets of Orinase, four tablets of Dymelor, two tablets of Diabinese, and two to three tablets of Tolinase.

DBI, which is not a sulfonylurea, is administered somewhat differently from the other drugs. Under no circumstances, even when the patient is being changed over from insulin, are large doses used initially. The rule with this drug seems to be: "Start low, go slow."

The reason for this is the incidence of nausea and vomiting which may develop, most likely at the higher dosage levels. Since these side effects may have serious consequences for the diabetic and because the reactions are highly individual, it is difficult to estimate in advance the safety of the higher dosage levels. Therefore, all diabetics who are given this drug are begun on the lowest possible dose which is gradually increased to the point where, consistent with drug safety, the diabetes is controlled.

There are some additional factors to be considered when the newly diagnosed diabetic is introduced to treatment. While such a patient will usually require the smallest dose, this is not always the case.

In exceptional instances, where the symptoms are pronounced or severe, the physician might decide it more appropriate to initiate therapy with the largest dose of sulfonylurea drug in order that control be established as quickly as possible. In effect, the treatment of any patient—new or old—will reflect the severity of the clinical picture. For this reason, while rules of treatment are essential, the therapy should be adjusted to the particular needs of the patient.

Where the diagnosis is incidental and the symptoms are mild, the patient will obviously be started with small doses of oral drugs. But where the onset of the disease has been explosive or the patient has many complaints, the physician may well prescribe initially larger doses of one or another sulfonylurea. As for DBI, even under these circumstances, treatment will begin with the smaller dose.

For the patient whose diabetes was discovered accidentally, perhaps during the course of a general physical examination, and who is free of symptoms, the use of an oral drug will offer several benefits.

It will help maintain control of the diabetes during periods of stress and overeating. In addition, there may be a long-term benefit for the patient in that the oral therapy could have the effect of slowing, or even stopping, what would otherwise be an inexorable progression of the disease. These patients may even be prevented from becoming insulin-dependent in later life.

The chart of available oral drugs on page 103 should prove useful for quick reference.

The choice of drug will be made by the physician on the basis of his estimation of the requirements of the disease as well as the needs of the patient.

From the standpoint of safety, Orinase has an unparalleled record.

From the standpoint of simplicity of treatment, Diabinese and Tolinase are outstanding because their long action often permits control of the dose with a single daily dose taken in the morning.

Dymelor, while apparently neither as safe as Orinase nor as easy or economical as Diabinese, is supposed to combine some features of both. However, since it and Tolinase are the newest oral drugs and there is only limited clinical experience as yet, more time is needed to evaluate them properly.

DBI has a narrow margin of safety and, unless the newer timed-disintegration (TD) capsules are used, a brief period of action. These TD capsules may be taken in a single or divided daily dose, depending upon need. The DBI tablets, however, usually have to be taken with each meal. While the daily dosage may range from two to eight tablets, three tablets, if tolerated without nausea and a metallic taste (signs of overdose), may be considered the average for safe use.

If the higher doses are needed to control the disease, great care should be exercised to assure that there are no untoward effects. Should the patient experience a metallic taste, nausea, or loss of appetite, he must immediately notify his physician and automatically reduce the dose.

In using DBI it should be understood that each patient dictates the maximum tolerable dose by his own individual response to the drug. Some patients cannot take two tablets a day without untoward effects, others can take as many as eight.

There are special hazards in the use of some oral drugs which should be taken into account. The prolonged action of Diabinese, for instance, while it provides certain advantages, also presents some danger to the atherosclerotic, mild diabetic in the older age group.

Among these patients, who tend to have a normal fasting blood sugar during sleep, the extended action of Diabinese into the night can provoke profound hypoglycemia. Consequently, this drug should be considered more appropriate for use in the younger more seriously diabetic patient who requires a larger dose than in the older patient whose disease is controlled with smaller doses.

If a patient, previously untreated with insulin, fails to show good results with one oral drug, success is still possible by changing to any one of the others. If each of the drugs fails singly, a combination of any of the sulfonylureas with DBI might still prove effective.

The diabetic who is being successfully treated

ORAL HYPOGLYCEMIC DRUGS

Trade Name	Generic Name	Type	Manufacturer	Size of Tablet	Daily Dose	Duration of Action
Orinase	tolbutamide	sulfonylurea	Upjohn	.5 gm (500 mg)	1 to 6 tablets (usually twice)	6 to 12 hours
Diabinese	chlorpropamide	sufonylurea	Pfizer	.1 gm (100 mg) .25 gm (250 mg)	100 to 500 mg	To 60 hrs.
Dymelor	acetohexamide	sulfonylurea	Lilly	.5 gm (500 mg)	1 to 4 tablets (once or twice)	12 to 24 hours
Tolinase	tolazimide	sulfonylurea	Upjohn	.1 gm (100 mg) .25 gm (250 mg)	100 to 750 mg	12 to 24 hours
DBI	phenformin	phenethylbiguanide	U.S. Vitamin & Pharm.	.025 gm (25 mg)	2 to 8 tablets (two or three times)	4 to 6 hours
DBI-TD	phenformin	phenethylbiguanide	U.S. Vitamin & Pharm.	.05 gm (50 mg) per capsule	1 to 4 capsules (once or twice)	8 to 12 hours

with oral medication may, under certain circumstances, have to be changed to insulin temporarily. This may take place during illness or infection; if some unusual stress produces a great metabolic strain; during surgery or, possibly, during pregnancy. In most of these cases, once the situation returns to normal, the patient can resume the oral drug.

However, should the diabetes itself change and assume a more severe form, the patient may have to make a permanent change from oral to insulin therapy.

Advantages of Oral Therapy

For the patient who takes an oral drug, life with diabetes is much easier than for the one who needs insulin.

This goes far beyond the obvious fact that it is easier to swallow a tablet than to plunge a hypodermic needle into one's skin every day. Wherever oral drugs work, they seem to provide better control over diabetes than does insulin. They leave the urine sugar-free without the danger of insulin shock.

Elimination of the hazard of shock is most important psychologically as well as physiologically. For the diabetic, it means release from a threat against which he must be on constant guard when taking insulin. He is relieved of the worry as well as the possible damage associated with shock.

And, of course, the actual business of living is vastly simplified by oral therapy. The insulin-treated diabetic, to avoid the possibility of shock, must adhere to a rigid eating schedule. If he misses or delays a meal, he faces the risk of shock. Similarly, if he overworks or even underworks, he may run into insulin or diabetic complications. None of this seems to be true for the patient who takes an oral drug. Somehow, this drug provides the diabetic with a new dimension of latitude in living.

The advantages of oral drugs extend beyond the realms of convenience and safety from insulin shock. Many diabetics, because of enfeeblement, advanced age, disease or some disability, are unable to give themselves injections and must have someone else do the job for them. In one case a son had to drive twenty miles every morning to give his mother the insulin injection she could not give herself.

Oral medication, on the other hand, eliminates this problem involving not only the diabetic but the son, the friend, the neighbor, or whoever it is who has to take time off every day to administer the injection.

There is also the matter of employability which is affected by insulin. Diabetics who take insulin frequently find that various ordinances may forbid their doing certain work. Because of the possibility of insulin shock, they are not permitted to drive public conveyances such as taxis, buses, or trains. But if they take oral drugs there is no danger of shock and they may drive any public conveyance.

Some diabetics who are allergic to sulfa drugs or to antibiotics may hesitate to change to a sulfonylurea through fear of possible allergy reactions. The fact is—and this bears repetition—that while the sufonylureas are remotely related to the sulfas, they are not true sulfas themselves and do not produce sulfa reactions. Nor are they antibiotics, therefore they do not produce antibiotic side effects. As for untoward reactions in the liver, kidneys, or blood, Orinase has not been known to produce any at all even in cases where it has been used eight years or more.

A further advantage is provided by the oral drug. We know that native insulin, produced in the islets of Langerhans, is carried by the blood directly from the pancreas to the liver, which seems to be its primary site of action. But injected insulin must make its way from the point of injection through the entire circulatory system before even part of it reaches its destination in the liver. On the way, much of it is trapped, blocked, and even destroyed by the action of various body substances.

Obviously, native insulin using the natural pathways to the liver is more effective than injected insulin that must go the long way around. The sulfonylureas, by working through the native insulin mechanism, seem to take advantage of this greater efficiency.

For the diabetic who is now freed from the daily need for an injection, the advantage of an oral drug is immediate and obvious. But the new drugs are having more far-reaching effects by spurring a new wave of diabetes research.

It is in this upsurge of scientific investigation, using them as research tools, that the greatest value of the new drugs may ultimately be found. For instance, experiments into the manner in which they work may provide a clue as to how insulin works. This, in turn, may offer a key to the mystery of diabetes itself—its cause or causes, and perhaps a possible cure.

CHAPTER 10

The Complications
of Diabetes

Today's diabetics, unlike those of half a century ago, can usually manage their disease with relative ease. Were it not for two major complications, they would have little to bother with apart from the ordinary steps involved in treatment. These complications—insulin shock and diabetic coma—do more than disturb the normal tenor of diabetes control. It is through them that diabetes can do its most serious damage.

Only the patient taking insulin is subject to insulin reaction and shock.

Diabetic coma, a hazard faced by all diabetics who allow the disease to get out of control, is more likely among those who are insulin-deficient.

Of the two complications, insulin reactions are more common and more sudden in onset. Diabetic coma is slow in onset and may take 24 hours or more to develop. But shock can literally happen in an instant. A diabetic may seem perfectly normal one moment, be unconscious the next.

For this reason, if a diabetic is ever uncertain as to whether any abnormal symptoms are due to insulin reaction or the development of coma, he should act at once to block insulin reaction. If he is wrong, he will have time to correct the error.

The Hazard of Insulin Reaction

Insulin reaction or *hypoglycemia,* is the result of too rapid and extreme a drop in blood-sugar. *This is caused by too much insulin activity.* Ordinarily, a normally healthy man has about a teaspoonful of sugar in his blood before breakfast. This rises slightly after each meal but is kept within a normal range by the insulin discharged by his pancreas. *At no time does his pancreas produce more insulin activity than is needed to keep his blood sugar at a normal level.*

A diabetic's blood-sugar level is higher than normal before breakfast and rises more than normally after each meal. Since the normal insulin supply cannot control this he must inject additional insulin. *This injected insulin does not match its activity to to the blood-sugar level as does the natural insulin produced in the body.*

Whenever a diabetic has *more* insulin activity than can be matched by the available blood sugar, the excess insulin produces such abnormally low blood-sugar levels that the brain and nervous system are deprived of an essential source of energy. The result is an insulin reaction which, if unchecked, can rapidly lead to shock.

Such a reaction might result from any of a number of situations which cause either too little blood-sugar or too much insulin activity.

A diabetic might miss a meal because of the rush of work; delay a meal to tend to a crying baby; fast during a Holy Day or skip a meal in preparation for Communion; become nauseated, vomit, have diarrhea—either from stomach upset, motion sickness, the taking of a purgative or emetic, an emotional upset, or some other cause; engage in unexpected physical activity such as playing some extra holes of golf or doing some hectic shopping in a crowded store.

All of these situations, by reducing the amount of available food or by using it up too swiftly, lower the level of blood sugar which the insulin dose is balanced to match. This brings about a relative excess of insulin and a raid into the body's *needed* store of sugar.

On the other side of this delicate balance, shock can be the product of simply too much insulin.

After many years of daily insulin injections, the process becomes so automatic and unthinking that a diabetic might measure an overdose without being aware of it. He might even forget that he has already taken an injection. Perhaps he was not fully awake or was thinking of something else at the time. So he takes another injection.

In all these cases the food intake and available blood sugar may be exactly as planned. The oversupply of insulin is what causes the trouble.

This about sums up the categories of things that could set the stage for an insulin reaction, but there is one special situation that deserves mention—drinking. For the diabetic, social drinking may sometimes be as perilous as extreme alcoholism.

This *does not* mean that the average adult with diabetes must abstain from alcohol for medical reasons. On the contrary, circumstances exist where alcohol is useful in diabetes. But it *does* mean that the diabetic who takes a drink must be particularly careful not to let his drinking unhinge his sense of time. The drink that makes a diabetic delay a meal is the drink too many. Nor is this the only potential danger.

A business associate invites a diabetic to have a drink after work. The diabetic agrees. He has a drink, then another. Even if he were not diabetic, several drinks would do something to his sense of time. Before he knows it, he has missed his train home and must wait for another.

By late afternoon, his insulin activity is reaching a peak. Maybe, if he is feeling no pain, he decides to have another drink. Maybe not. In any case, whether he realizes it or not, he is missing the meal he should be eating to accommodate the insulin in his system.

He begins to sweat, feels a little dizzy perhaps. It might be the liquor. So he leaves his friend and goes out into the air. Perhaps he decides it is time to try again for the train. Meanwhile the insulin, hungry for sugar, deprives his nervous system and cerebral cortex of this vital energy source.

Suddenly, in the street, he staggers and collapses, struck down by insulin shock. A well-meaning passer-by bends over to help, smells the alcohol on his breath, shrugs and moves on. No point getting mixed up with a drunk.

Because his collapse is mistaken for drunkenness, the underlying insulin shock may be undetected and untreated long enough to cause irreparable damage.

Even without the smell of liquor on a diabetic's breath, the symptoms of insulin reaction often look enough like drunkenness to make a mistake all too easy. This makes it more important for the diabetic to carry a card, easily accessible, identifying him as a diabetic and describing what to do in emergencies.

He should also let his friends, neighbors, associates, classmates, and teachers know he is diabetic. Diabetics, especially adolescent girls and young women, frequently try to keep their ailment a secret, thus adding to their own difficulties in an emergency.

Finally, the diabetic—as well as those associated with him—should know the symptoms of insulin reaction and be able to recognize them promptly and treat them.

How to Recognize and Correct Insulin Reaction

The first sign of an insulin reaction is usually mild hunger. Then, in order, come

> sweating
> dizziness
> palpitation
> pale, moist skin

If the reaction is untreated, these symptoms follow:

> shallow breathing
> trembling
> blurred or double vision
> mental confusion and disorientation
> very strange behavior (disrobing or something equally odd)
> finally, the end symptom, loss of consciousness

At any point before unconsciousness sets in, taking a lump of sugar, a piece of candy, drinking soda pop, fruit juice or anything else containing sugar can abolish the symptoms swiftly.

There is hardly anything in all of medicine as dramatic as the almost instantaneous correction of insulin reaction after the administration of sugar. That is why the diabetic on insulin should always carry an emergency supply of hard candy or lump sugar. Within 30 seconds or a minute after the sugar is swallowed there is a complete return to normality with, oddly enough, no memory of what took place after the start of mental confusion.

Recovery is not so prompt for the diabetic whose insulin reaction is untreated until he is already unconscious. In that case it may be 15 minutes before recovery becomes apparent, and the diabetic may be left with a headache.

If left untreated for too long, the reaction may be so severe that the diabetic cannot swallow candy or sugar. In that case, a doctor should be called at once. He should also be called if the patient does not respond to treatment.

If possible, glucagon should be administered by hypodermic as an emergency measure. Glucagon ampoules are part of the necessary equipment for all insulin-sensitive diabetics. The doctor, when he arrives, will probably administer glucose in order to raise the blood sugar with the least possible delay.

The longer the patient is unconscious before treatment begins, the slower and less complete will be the recovery.

It is important for every diabetic and everyone close to him to remember that repeated and prolonged incidents of insulin reaction can have cumulative effects. Therefore, they must be avoided or, if they do occur, treated the instant they are *suspected*. The diabetic who feels a growing hunger or thinks he is perspiring should never wait to see if the symptoms will go away by themselves—no matter how mild they seem.

The *first suspicion*, however slight, should be treated without delay as a full onset of insulin reaction. Where insulin reaction is concerned, the diabetic must take absolutely no chances. It is far better to take emergency sugar unnecessarily than to risk shock.

There is a wide variety of sugars and sweets that can help a diabetic overcome insulin reaction. These include sugar, fruit juices, sweetened drinks, syrups, soda pop, honey, jams and jellies, and candies.

Artificial sweeteners and sugar substitutes are absolutely useless and must *never* be used in these cases. This applies to the so-called diabetic candies, jellies, jams, and similar products. These may be fine in the ordinary diabetic diet where sugar is being avoided. But in the event of an insulin reaction *real* sugar is essential.

Whole fresh fruit, bread, or other starches are of no immediate value, since they are too slowly digested to compensate for an acute sugar shortage. The diabetic in shock should not be given too much sugar too rapidly or he may become nauseated.

It is better to administer a lump of sugar or a glass of fruit juice. Then, as his mental powers recover, give him a bit more. The important thing is the speed with which the sugar is given, not the amount. After the patient has emerged from the reaction, he should be given some regular nourishment—fruit, bread, or other high-carbohydrate food—to provide a reserve of sugar for later use.

Before leaving the subject of insulin reaction, it would be wise to emphasize once more the importance of recognizing and treating this condition at once. If a diabetic feels poorly in any way or behaves strangely, *he should be treated for insulin reaction immediately—even if the symptoms are doubtful or do not follow a regular pattern.*

Relatives, friends, and others who are close to the diabetic should be ready to act the instant he shows any deviation from normal behavior.

The teacher should be careful to note inattention on the part of the normally attentive diabetic student.

The wife or associate should suspect that a rise of irritability or temper is a sign of insulin reaction rather than real anger.

The Hazard of Diabetic Coma

Coma, the second major complication of diabetes, is the exact opposite of insulin shock. Shock begins with an abnormal drop in blood sugar due to *too much insulin activity*. Coma develops from an abnormal rise in blood sugar due to *too little insulin activity*.

The development of coma follows the same pattern as untreated diabetes. Lacking insulin activity with which to metabolize sugar, the body hungrily raids its own fat and protein tissue for substitute energy sources. This brings about a rise of ketone and acetone in the blood; then, as the normally alkaline blood becomes loaded with these fatty acids, acidosis and coma follow.

Unlike insulin reaction, diabetic coma is slow and undramatic in its onset. It is also relatively infrequent today. Yet before the discovery of insulin, many adult and practically all juvenile diabetics eventually died in coma.

The symptoms of diabetic coma are identical with those of severe diabetes:

> Frequent, copious urination
> Constant thirst
> Persistent hunger
> Flushed, dry skin
> Weakness, fatigue and drowsiness
> Fruity odor of breath
> Deep, labored breathing
> Vomiting
> And finally, unconsciousness

The events leading to coma can be set into motion by any of a wide variety of events.

A patient might be taking drugs which raise the level of blood sugar, such as ACTH, cortisone or its derivatives, or certain diuretics which are commonly used to rid the body of excess fluids.

An insulin-treated patient may neglect or delay his injections.

A patient using oral drugs may forget to take the tablets.

There might be errors of insulin administration.

A diabetic might use a syringe with the wrong markings and thus take too little insulin.

He might take the wrong insulin or a less concentrated insulin. By mistakenly using U40 instead of U80 insulin, he would be getting only half the activity he needs.

He might use insulin that is too old or has been spoiled by freezing or overheating.

He might not mix properly an insulin vial that requires mixing—Protamine Zinc, NPH, or Lente.

He might even become involved in something that absorbs his attention and, because insulin injections become unthinkingly routine, imagine that he took it when actually he had not.

These and similar lapses in diabetes control are *external* factors which may precipitate coma by providing less insulin activity than the diabetic normally needs.

There are also *internal* factors that may increase the diabetic's need for insulin above that provided by the usual dose. This can happen in a number of ways—some subtle, some obvious.

As a diabetic grows older he needs less food. If he does not reduce his food intake to match his reduced need, then he will require more insulin. Even if his diabetes had been mild enough to be controlled by diet alone this may change the nature of his ailment so that a need for insulin develops.

Illness, injury, a decline in physical activity, and various other situations that arise in the course of daily living may result in an increased need for insulin. If unsatisfied, the process leading to diabetic coma is set into motion.

A diabetic catches cold and goes to bed. Because of the decline in physical activity he may need 10 to 12 percent more insulin to handle the sugar which would otherwise have been used up by work, exercise or getting about. If he does not take the extra insulin, in about 24 hours he may have high blood sugar; and the symptoms of diabetes will begin to show themselves almost as though the disease were untreated. Ketosis will follow, then acidosis and, finally, coma. But all this will develop gradually, and with the cushion of time providing a safety factor, the situation should be recognized and corrected before any damage is done.

Just as diabetic coma takes longer to develop than insulin shock, so the response to treatment is equally slow. Insulin reactions are reversed in a matter of seconds when sugar is administered. The trend to coma may take hours to rectify.

Factors That Influence Coma

Gradual though the onset of coma may be, the rate at which it develops is variable, with three factors influencing the tempo.

First, there is the age of the patient. The process is faster in children because they have less sugar stored in the liver than adults and their metabolic needs for growth and energy are higher. Therefore, the raiding of body fat and protein proceeds at a more rapid pace than in adults. In children, the whole process from original insulin deficiency through ketosis, acidosis and on to actual coma may speed up and take only a day.

Second, there is the nature of the provocation. A cold will not have the same impact on insulin need as will pneumonia. A minor cut will not be as provocative as a multiple fracture. An error in dose will not be as important as failing to take insulin altogether.

Finally, there is the nature of the diabetes. An insulin-deficient diabetic is obviously more susceptible to coma than a maturity-onset diabetic who does produce some natural insulin and is not as dependent upon an outside source. In the latter, internal stress is not as catastrophic and the possibility of an insulin shortage not so serious.

From this standpoint, an attack of lobar pneumonia might be more serious for a young adult diabetic than for an older diabetic. The young adult, with a higher insulin need, would develop ketosis relatively easily. The older diabetic with a slight insulin need, or treating his disease with oral drugs or diet, would have no great problem and might not go into ketosis at all.

Nevertheless, the stress of illness or injury so disturbs the balance of the body that the diabetic who normally can control his disease with only diet or oral therapy may develop a need for insulin during the course of the disturbance. When the provocation is removed, he may return to his usual treatment. All this, of course, is carefully controlled by the physician.

Treatment of Coma

In its early stages, the onset of diabetic coma may be treated at home unless it is complicated by other factors that require hospitalization. The mild-to-moderate ketosis with which the trend to coma begins can be recognized by the symptoms of excessive thirst, frequent urination and a feeling of being "not quite right."

As soon as these symptoms appear the diabetic should rest and avoid any physical activity.

He should test his urine for sugar and acetone.

He should report to his doctor by telephone and, thereafter until the situation is cleared up, should test every urine voided for both sugar and acetone.

If his urine test shows sugar and acetone, he should immediately take an injection of quick-acting regular insulin. In severe diabetes the dose should be 30 to 40 units; in milder cases, 15 to 20 units.

If the urine test shows acetone but no sugar, the diabetic must take candy, honey, sugar, or a sweet drink as well as the insulin injection. This is more common among juvenile diabetics with a low sugar reserve than among adults. The purpose of the sugar is to provide a buffer against the possibility of insulin reaction and to furnish glucose instead of fat as an energy source.

In any case, the diabetic in ketosis should also drink a glass of fruit juice or tea sweetened with 3 teaspoons of sugar every one or two hours.

The same dose of regular insulin should be repeated every two or three hours until the urine is free of acetone. At this time the fruit juice or sweetened drinks may be discontinued and the normal meal schedule resumed.

If the urine tests show high sugar levels even though there is no acetone present; or if the original symptoms persist despite the disappearance of acetone from the urine, the injections of regular insulin should continue at the same intervals, but with only half the original dose. They should be stopped only when the patient feels normal again and his urine is free of sugar.

If the ketosis symptoms are more severe than those mentioned above; should extreme nausea, vomiting, drowsiness, or deep, labored breathing occur, then hospital treatment is probably needed. In any case, the physician should be notified at once.

Although both of the major complications of diabetes arise from opposite causes and require different treatments, they are sometimes confused with one another. For this reason, we will compare their characteristics and show how they can be told apart.

Insulin Reaction	*Diabetic Coma*
Sudden onset	Slow, gradual onset
Perspiration, pale skin	Dry, hot skin
Dizziness	No dizziness
Palpitation	No palpitation
Hunger	No hunger
Normal urination	Excessive urination
Normal thirst	Excessive thirst
Shallow breathing	Deep, labored breathing
Normal breath odor	Fruity breath odor
Confusion, disorientation, strange behavior	Drowsiness and great lethargy
Urinary sugar absent or slight	Large amounts of urinary sugar
No acetone in urine	Acetone present in urine

By checking these symptoms, it should be fairly easy to distinguish between insulin reaction and diabetic coma. But, if there is any doubt at all, the diabetic should be treated for insulin reaction until a fuller diagnosis is available. The speed of insulin reaction allows no time for delay or error. The slowness of diabetic coma, on the other hand, does grant time for the correction of an error.

Whatever the complication, the physician should be notified at once. The fact that an insulin reaction may be quickly corrected by swallowing a piece of candy, or that ketosis might be eliminated by an injection of regular insulin in no way removes the possibility of danger. The underlying reason for the complication remains to be determined and corrected. That task belongs to the physician.

By curbing the major complications of diabetes—reducing their incidence and correcting them promptly when they do appear—the diabetic may be better able to cope with other ailments which often accompany the disease.

The most common of these is arteriosclerosis or hardening of the arteries. This is a common companion of aging even among non-diabetics, but it frequently appears somewhat earlier in diabetics.

Exactly why certain processes linked with aging should speed up with diabetes is not yet known. Nor does this situation seem to be affected by the quality of diabetes management. Nevertheless, the patient's ability to meet the stresses and strains of daily living as well as the wear and tear of aging can only be enhanced by intelligent care and good control.

What Is Good Control of Diabetes?

The question of what constitutes good control of diabetes is, to put it mildly, open to some discussion. Perhaps "argument" would be a better word to describe the disagreement between the school of the sugar-free urine and the school which disregards urinary sugar.

The sugar-free school reaches all the way back to the pre-insulin past in its insistence upon rigid control to the point of deprivation.

The other view, expounded by Dr. Edward Tolstoi of the New York Hospital, holds that the presence of *some* sugar in the urine *without* the usual symptoms of diabetes is desirable because "it protects the patient from overdoses of insulin and consequent insulin reactions."

The best control of diabetes, which would permit the diabetic to live as normally as possible while offering the best protection from complications, lies somewhere between these opposing views.

Rigid insistence on sugar-free urine, while it may protect the diabetic from coma, does expose him to a lowered sugar reserve and possible insulin reaction. Child diabetics, whose sugar reserves are naturally low and whose insulin-sugar balance is subject to unpredictable change, cannot maintain a sugar-free urine without teetering on the brink of insulin reaction.

On the other hand, where a sugar-free urine poses no great danger—as in moderate, stable diabetes— the diabetic who has no sugar in the urine *feels better* than one who has some sugar. And the more sugar there is present, the less well he feels. Furthermore, the presence of *unnecessary* sugar may bring the diabetic too close to the slope leading to ketosis, acidosis, and coma.

For these reasons, best control is probably achieved when the following criteria are met:

The diabetic feels well.

His diet permits him to maintain normal weight and provides all the nutritional requirements for growth, work, play, and the regular activities of daily living.

Just enough treatment, whether it be insulin, oral therapy, or dietary restriction, is used to assure proper utilization of the foods eaten without provoking insulin reaction or coma.

The treatment is simplified to the point where the diabetic can live and work with the absolute minimum of interference from the needs of the ailment.

Wherever possible, the diabetic tries to maintain a sugar-free urine or one with the smallest possible amount of sugar.

For about 20 percent of all diabetics—those who are sensitive to insulin and whose disease is unstable, sugar-free urine is impossible. In those cases, moderate amounts of urinary sugar cannot be avoided without running the risk of insulin reaction.

Where these criteria of treatment are met, and there is sufficient flexibility to adjust to whatever changes may occur, then the diabetic has his disease under good control.

Steering a course between excess and insufficient insulin activity, he should then be able to reduce the danger of complications to an absolute minimum while feeling well, working well and living well.

Short of eliminating the diabetes entirely, this is the substantial best that any treatment can seek to accomplish.

PART THREE

The Problems of Diabetes

CHAPTER 11

The Diabetic Child

It is said that when a child develops diabetes the doctor immediately has two patients—the child and the mother.

This is an understatement.

The diagnosis of diabetes in a child frequently sends out waves of stress which reach far beyond the immediate family.

Not only are the child and mother affected, but so are the father, the other children, in-laws and relatives, friends, and sometimes even teachers. And all these, by their reactions, in turn may affect the child and his attitude toward the disease.

Diabetes in a child is fraught with emotion for the parents and is difficult for them to accept with equanimity. Since there is a possibility of heredity factors being involved, unconscious guilt may assail them. Some even take the attitude that this is a punishment visited upon them from above. Furthermore, the day-in, day-out routine of urine tests, injections, and special eating schedules are chores which the mother must perform; and they are no easy matter to cope with at first.

The mother may react by rejecting the child and treating him with harsh rigidity. She may do the exact opposite and become doting, overprotective, and indulgent. In either case, the child's adjustment to the disease is bound to suffer.

Relatives, especially grandparents, can be very harmful to a child's morale if their reactions are tinged with overanxiety and hysteria. The best intentions of the physician are often thwarted by these attitudes of parents, grandparents and other relatives.

Teachers may be overly disturbed by a child's diabetes and treat him with marked difference from the other children. This is bound to impede the child.

Finally, if there are other children in the family, they are likely to be affected by the situation and, in turn, produce an effect. Depending upon their own security and adjustment, they may tend to resent the special attention given to the diabetic child. The patient, on his part, could easily come to resent the fact that he is suffering the pain of injection and the deprivation of certain foods while the other children are not.

In the face of this downpour of problems, how is the diabetic child ever to achieve proper adjustment to a disease with which he must live the rest of his days? There is no easy, precisely defined answer to this question.

Yet there *is* an answer—one that can be found only in the love and intuitive understanding of the parents.

No normal parents can be expected to accept diabetes in a child casually. But, if they are to help the child, they should place the emphasis on the child rather than on the disease.

This means that they should first accept the child as a human being. The fact that this is a child with diabetes—as it may be a child with any other ailment—is of secondary importance.

The parents should also try to provide a home atmosphere that is relaxed and tranquil, one in which the father as well as the mother plays a positive role. The father's participation in the activities and thought of the child is particularly important and will help provide an additional measure of stability and security. All this will fortify the child, help him withstand the misunderstandings and blunders of overanxious, hysterical, or uninformed outsiders.

How Parents Can Help Diabetic Child

Apart from these general rules, there are some specific suggestions which will help parents—and the child—to achieve a better adjustment to the disease: The parents should become intelligently informed about diabetes; disregard the mysticism, mumbo-jumbo and old-wives' tales and seek out the latest scientific information. They should avoid being either overrestrictive or overindulgent. They should avoid bribery, cajolery, or intimidation to make the child accept injections and other necessities of treatment. They should accept the fact, and try to have the child accept the fact, that the injections, while painful, are necessary. The same applies to such deprivations as denial of certain foods and activities. They should try to treat the disease in such a way that it *seems* to cause the least visible disruption in everyday living. The regular living habits of the family should go on as before. The other children should be treated exactly the same as before, allowed to eat the same, play the same, have the same rights.

By following these suggestions it should be possible for the parents to establish a situation in which the diabetic child has a maximum feeling of security as an individual and as a member of the family. The closer this ideal is approached, the better will be the child's attitude toward his disease; and the fewer will be the strains set up within the family.

The nature of "juvenile diabetes" has already been discussed in the chapter, The Development of Diabetes.

As we know, it erupts dramatically and is usually associated with one or more of the infections so common in childhood. Most often, the child diabetic is already suffering from acute acidosis when the diabetes is recognized, and requires immediate hospitalization. For any child this will be a traumatic experience, but the stronger his sense of security, the better he usually weathers it.

Diabetes Is Bewildering Experience for Child

When the child leaves the hospital and returns home, the whole world seems topsy-turvy. The disease is incomprehensible to him and the attitude he develops will be determined by the attitude and behavior of his parents.

He will discover that he must have at least one injection of insulin a day.

He must have his urine tested for sugar and acetone twice each day, before breakfast and before the evening meal.

He must eat six times a day—three meals and three snacks—at prescribed times and with clock-sure regularity.

His diet is no longer subject to his whim as before—he cannot normally eat sugar, candy, syrups, and soda pop—although he must eat enough of the properly balanced foods to provide for proper growth.

It might be wise here for parents to understand that rapidly absorbed sugars, such as candy, pop, and the like, cause a sharp rise in blood-sugar levels, and a dumping of sugar into the urine whereby it is passed out of the body. This represents wasted eating. On the other hand, these same rapidly absorbed sugars can be very useful in checking insulin reaction where a rapid rise in blood sugar is needed.

The child diabetic, in addition to injections, urine tests and a rigidly timed eating schedule, must also face certain restrictions on his physical activity. If his insulin action reaches a peak at 3 o'clock, his mother may no longer allow him out in the street to play with the other children at that time, unless he has a snack first. She knows, although he will not, that peak insulin activity coinciding with violent physical activity can result in an insulin reaction.

These changes and restrictions in his mode of life will be beyond the understanding of the young diabetic child. The whole idea of diabetes will be almost impossible for him to grasp, no matter how diligently the parents try to explain. Nevertheless, the young child will usually accept the injections, tests, and restrictions as part of the incomprehensible, inconvenient, and often painful rule imposed on him by the adult world. It is only as he grows older and approaches adolescence that he will begin to question. When this happens, a new set of problems will arise.

Odd Characteristics of Childhood Diabetes

Childhood diabetes has some peculiar characteristics for which the parents should be well prepared.

The first of these can be truly shocking.

About two months or so after the child's disease is diagnosed and treatment begun, there is frequently a dramatic improvement. The symptoms of the disease vanish, the insulin has to be discontinued and the child seems miraculously cured—almost as though the parents' prayers have been answered.

Unfortunately, this is a caprice of the disease. Parents should recognize it as just that, rather than let their hopes be raised, then dashed as the diabetes flares up again permanently, which it inevitably does.

There is another characteristic of childhood diabetes against which parents should be on guard. Up until about the age of ten, an insulin reaction is often accompanied by symptoms usually associated with the opposite complication—acidosis. These symptoms are vomiting and headache.

Unless the parents are aware of this quirk of the disease and *treat immediately for insulin reaction,* serious error is likely to result.

Even where acidosis *is* the complication involved, *the child who vomits will need sugar along with insulin.*

Treating the Diabetic Child

Ordinarily, the problems of the pre-school diabetic are relatively few, since he is prone to accept parental authority and his environment is more amenable to control. It is easier for a mother to watch over the physical activity and mealtimes of a pre-school child than of a child who spends a large part of the time away from home.

At this stage, the treatment is mainly administered by the parent, who does the testing, gives the injections, regulates eating and, to a lesser degree, physical activity.

Good treatment for a diabetic child generally consists of an adequate diet that permits full growth and enough insulin so that the child can utilize most of the food eaten. Except for the restrictions on concentrated sugars, the diabetic child's diet should be the same in calories and nutrients as that of any normal child his age.

Because of the diabetic child's high sensitivity to insulin, a sugar-free urine may lead to frequent incidents of insulin reaction. So some urinary sugar is permissible at various times during the day. If the morning test shows *no* sign of urinary acetone, control of the child's diabetes is usually good if the child is also growing properly.

Should the child wet the bed, have to urinate frequently or become excessively thirsty, he probably needs a larger dose of long-acting insulin.

The administration of insulin may be one of the most important problems at the outset. There is pain involved and the appearance of the hypodermic syringe is not particularly reassuring. So the child might become frightened and resist the injection.

The parent should try to keep the injection simple and uncomplicated. The syringe should be prepared and the dose measured out of the young child's sight at first. Then the injection should be given with as little fuss as possible.

If the child feels extreme pain, the injection might best be given in the buttocks, which are less sensitive to pain. In extreme cases, the child's resistance might be so great that he will have to be held in order to receive the injection.

Some parents make the mistake of bribing or cajoling the child into accepting the injection. This spoils the child, creates a situation in which he can use the injection as a means of blackmail. Other parents may threaten or scold if the child resists the injection. This will only make him less cooperative later on.

If the child has a normally good adjustment and is accepted, and if the parents are intelligent and understanding, the chances are that the injection will not create too great a problem.

Still, generalizations are always dangerous, particularly so in diabetes. Where injection difficulties arise, the parents should try to ease the situation, keeping one fact firmly in mind: *Whatever the circumstances, the insulin injection must be given in the proper dosage at the proper time.*

In order to prevent the development of problems later in the child's life, it is important for the parent not to be overprotective. As soon as possible, depending upon the age, character and intelligence of of the child, there should be a gradual shifting of responsibility for the management of the disease.

Teaching the Child to Treat Himself

The average diabetic child of five can and should be taught to test his own urine for sugar and acetone. This might be done easily by pretending that it is a sort of game. No reading or calculations are involved, only a simple procedure and the matching of colors.

Gradually, after the child has come to accept the injection, the parent can change the sites to include the arms and thighs so the child can see how it is done and, as he develops the ability, be encouraged to do it himself.

By the time the child is eight or nine, he should be taught how to measure his own insulin, prepare and sterilize the syringe.

At about twelve or thirteen, the child ought to be able to take over full responsibility for the management of the disease. He should handle his tests, his injections, watch his diet and activity schedule, be able to detect and control such complications as insulin reaction and acidosis.

Probably the most serious problem of childhood diabetes is the recognition of these complications. The young child is frequently unable to recognize the warning signs of insulin reaction or acidosis. During the excitement of a game, even a passive one, he may disregard the fact that he is perspiring. On the other extreme, he may be too absorbed in other matters to relate the fact that he is urinating frequently.

Sometimes an intelligent child may devise his own approach to the detection of complications. One bright boy of five was able to recognize what he called "a shaky funny feeling." Whenever he had that feeling he knew he had to take something sweet—usually some candy he carried for such an emergency—and come home for a snack.

Until the child is old enough to detect the symptoms of complications—and even afterwards—the parents, teachers, friends and playmates should be alert for such signs as excessive perspiration, trembling, inattention, irritation or temper in the case of insulin reaction; unusual thirst, frequent urination, weakness or lethargy in the case of acidosis.

Frequently, complications may set in while the child is asleep. For this reason, a parent should, from time to time, pass a hand over the sleeping child's forehead for any sign of perspiration that cannot be attributed to humidity or temperature. A clammy forehead would indicate an insulin reaction, and the child should be given fruit juice or a piece of candy.

On the other hand, a hot, dry forehead, bedwetting or frequent nocturnal trips to the toilet warn of impending ketosis and the need for an injection of 5 or 10 units of regular insulin *plus the feeding of something sweet such as fruit juice.*

Problems of Childhood Diabetes

Because of the extreme instability of juvenile diabetes, many seemingly ordinary things such as season of the year, weather and temperature, may create problems affecting the child's need for insulin. Playing out of doors on a bright, sunny day may reduce his need for insulin. If heavy rains keep him indoors, his physical activity is reduced, causing an increase in insulin need.

When the season and weather permit more physical activity, less insulin is usually needed. Where there is less physical activity more insulin is needed.

In some of the special camps for diabetic children, during rainy weather the children exercise indoors on treadmills to obtain the physical activity they would otherwise miss.

Diabetes does not create serious social problems for the pre-school child. But once the child leaves the shelter of the home to begin his formal education, social as well as new physical problems appear.

The first of these involves integrating the classroom schedule with the child's eating habits. This should not create too great a difficulty if the parents understand that the child's insulin doses and meal schedule may be manipulated to provide an individual adjustment to any new situation.

The type or dose of insulin may be changed to fit the child's new eating program. Similarly, the child's food schedule may be altered to match the insulin activity.

Many children usually need a small dose of quick-acting regular insulin along with a larger dose of slower, long-acting insulin (NPH, Lente, etc.). The regular insulin acts only in the four hours between breakfast and lunch. The long-acting insulin works for the rest of the day.

If the school schedule delays the child's lunch, a reduction in the regular insulin may be necessary to avoid the possibility of insulin reaction. Regular insulin should also be reduced if the child has frequent insulin reactions between breakfast and lunch. On the other hand, if he spills sugar or urinates frequently during that period, regular insulin should be increased.

Similarly, eating schedules can also be modified to meet the needs of living. A child who normally takes the mid-day meal at 12:00 registers for kindergarten and has to start school at noon. This makes it necessary for him to have the noon meal earlier, say at 11:00, so that he can get to school on time. Since this would mean a longer period without food in the early afternoon and a resulting drop in blood sugar, the child may compensate with a heavier than normal snack at his 3 o'clock eating time.

Strange problems often arise. One particularly bright student who was especially good in arithmetic started a new term by going into an arithmetic slump. His marks were high in every subject but, for some reason, he could not seem to get anywhere with arithmetic.

His doctor heard about it during a routine examination, became suspicious and questioned the boy closely. It turned out that the boy's schedule for the new term was so set up that he had his arithmetic class just before lunch and right after the gymnasium period.

The spurt of physical activity in gymnasium depleted his carbohydrate reserve. When he went into his arithmetic class he was on the threshold of insulin reaction and simply could not concentrate. Then he went to lunch, restored his carbohydrate and finished the rest of the school day with his normal intelligence at full power.

Once the cause for the arithmetic slump was discovered it was easy to correct. A sweet snack at the end of the gymnasium period restored his blood-sugar; and his arithmetic marks rose accordingly.

As the growing child moves out of the home, special alertness is needed to recognize situations of potential conflict between the needs of the diabetes and the requirements of the environment. One way or another, it should be possible to make some sort of accommodation so that the child will be able to function as normally as possible.

Lunches are a common problem for diabetic children. If they eat in the school cafeterias they are usually fed high-carbohydrate meals. While normally quite nourishing, these represent a certain amount of wasted eating for the child who cannot utilize certain carbohydrates as well as other children. For this reason he would be better nourished if he brought his lunch from home—food high in proteins such as meats, fish, eggs, or cheeses, which he can use without waste.

As the child gets older, changes in living patterns bring inevitable changes in the problems of treatment. The child begins to go to bed later, he stays out and plays longer. These and similar developments are bound to demand changes and adjustments in the insulin as well as in the eating schedule.

It is when the diabetic child starts going to school that he will—if he hasn't before—begin to feel that faint stirring of social problems; a realization that he is somehow different from the other children.

During the lunch recess, his classmates may cluster around the "Good Humor" man outside and soon they will all be eating ice cream. All, that is, but the diabetic child. He, for reasons he is probably unable to understand fully, will have to exercise self-discipline and refuse to share in the fun. Not that he can't have ice cream. He can—but only at certain stipulated times within his schedule. But the other children can have their ice cream any time—and as often as they like.

In childhood there is also the flood of birthday parties, becoming more numerous as the child's circle of friends expands. At these parties there is the usual gorging of ice cream, chocolates, layer cake, and other goodies washed down by various kinds of soda pop. The children have a wonderful time stuffing themselves—all but the child diabetic. He must not indulge. He is different.

If the timing of the party happens to coincide with the child's snack time, the mother might be able to make some adjustment so that the child could have ice cream or cookies during the party. This may help to ease the situation, but it will not entirely remove the mounting sense of "difference."

It is at this stage that the child's feeling of acceptance within the family begins to assume great importance in the diabetes picture. Sparks of rebellion and noncooperation are bound to show as he approaches adolescence. But whether they burst hotly into flame will be greatly influenced by the child's attitude toward his parents—and their attitude toward him.

Both overindulgence and neglect, while they do their damage to the child, are rooted in the personality and adjustment problems of the parents. To correct them, intelligence and human understanding are more important than medical understanding.

But rigid restriction of a child often *can* be corrected by improved medical understanding.

Outmoded Beliefs May Endanger Child

Many doctors, practicing today, retain a number of the old-fashioned attitudes about diabetes. Some even cling to the conviction that diabetes can best be treated by deprivation. These attitudes are passed along to the parents as medical gospel. A situation of rigid control is created, and the child is ultimately bound to rebel, sometimes at considerable damage to himself.

What is more, rigid control is *not* the best control, since it usually increases the incidence of insulin reactions. Children who are allowed only three precisely measured meals a day without extra snacks to compensate for peaks of physical activity are bound to have insulin reactions. Any attempt to correct this situation by decreasing the insulin dose rather than by increasing the flexibility of the food allowance adds a new set of dangers, since the child's insulin needs must invariably grow as he grows.

It is up to the parents to exercise intelligence. They must learn where to establish a balance between the actual needs imposed by the disease and the needs of the child as a human being. They must also be able to draw a line between practices established by medical knowledge and dogmas handed down by custom.

Some parents still believe that everything sweet is dangerous and do not allow their children ice cream or other sweets which *are* permissible, say, as a three-o'clock snack.

There is one particular misconception which can create a vast number of problems by adding to the existing restrictions on the child's life. This is the belief that children with diabetes are more susceptible to infection than others.

This is not true. The juvenile or young adult diabetic who takes insulin is no more prone to infection than anyone else. Cuts, wounds, bruises, and fractures heal just as rapidly and as well as with non-diabetics. It is only with the approach of late middle age that the balance changes.

Parents often wonder whether or not they should send the child to a diabetic camp for the summer holiday.

The answer to this depends upon the child and his adjustment to the disease. If the child has not adjusted to the diabetes, if he feels isolated or unique, if he seems overly dependent in handling his urine tests and other chores, then a diabetic camp might be very helpful.

It will bring him into contact with other diabetics and thus reduce his feeling of isolation. It will teach him to test his urine, take his insulin and generally make him better able to manage his disease.

For the child with a good attitude toward his disease, a diabetic camp is not advised. Instead he would be better off in a regular camp with his everyday friends where he would learn, as he must, to function in a non-diabetic world.

The diabetic child, even one whose treatment is relatively flexible and whose family adjustment is on the highest level, will show signs of resentment and rebellion as he grows older. He will discover that his urine tests do not immediately show a rise in sugar even if he takes a forbidden chocolate or eats a helping of ice cream on the sly. At other times, his sugar may rise even though he has had absolutely no extras.

All this will make him question the validity of the restrictions—and he will begin to violate them, striving as far as possible to do the things other children are permitted to do. If the parent-child relationship is a good one, this rebellion should not get out of hand and will probably be amenable to adjustment. If the relationship is a bad one or the treatment has been too rigid, the rebellion could persist with serious consequences.

A doctor of the old school, who believed in rigid control, treated a number of child diabetics at a noted Midwestern clinic. Each week the children reported for examination and, as part of the practice, presented carefully kept charts showing the results of the urine tests they gave themselves daily.

One of the patients, a pretty young lady of about 10, showed remarkably good control, and her urine charts were invariably excellent as far as sugar and acetone were concerned. On the basis of general health and growth as well as the showing of the urine tests, her progress was so good that the doctor took understandable pride in the excellence of his treatment.

One day the young lady appeared for examination. When the doctor asked for her urine chart she started to hand it over then abruptly pulled it back. "Oh, no," she blurted, "that's next week's chart. Here's this week's."

The doctor was so shocked that his belief in his treatment was shattered. The girl had obviously broken his restrictive rules, had been eating foods forbidden to her and had then falsified her test charts to cover up her rebellion. Despite this, her physical condition seemed fine and she was showing all of the appearances of good control. There was nothing the doctor could do to restore his position—either in his own eyes or in the girl's.

This anecdote is not intended to prove that the child who rebels against restrictions and flagrantly violates a regimen will be better off for it. On the contrary.

But it does show that urine tests are not always true, that, even when true, they are not always an accurate reflection of the diabetes situation; and that a certain amount of dietary leeway is possible without irreparable damage being done.

Revolt against authority is part of the normal process of growing up. In the diabetic child, it has an additional spur. The intelligent parent must understand this, anticipate it and be prepared to compensate for it with additional insulin or whatever else might be indicated.

About the best that can be hoped for is to have the rebellion minimized and kept within bounds. This goal can best be attained where the family relationships are good and where the treatment is balanced between the needs of the ailment and the human needs of the child.

CHAPTER 12

The Diabetic Adolescent

Adolescence is a time of great change and upheaval. Diabetes acquired in this period is the juvenile form with its explosive onset and tendency toward ketosis.

Diabetic or not, the adolescent grows at a prodigious rate, and the total need for calories is greater than at any other time of life. Equally great is the expenditure of calories to fill the vast demand for energy.

Adolescence is also a time when the activity of the endocrine glands is at its peak. The dynamic changes begun at puberty rise to a crescendo and involve the pituitary, the thyroid, the adrenal, and other glands.

Emotionally, the adolescent swings wildly between childhood and adulthood. There is great instability as the personality seeks to adjust itself. It is a period of touchiness and sensitivity, of resentment and rebellion against the controls imposed upon the child by the adult world. The adolescent is in constant battle to assert himself and to win the right to make his own decisions regarding his life—and the only way this is ultimately done is by casting off parental control.

The problems of adolescence produce great conflicts both within the adolescent himself and also with his environment. This is true for all youngsers who have stopped being children but are not yet adults. Not only do they break with the past, they must also find the future—and this is almost always beset with questions, fears and uncertainties.

Physical Problems of Diabetic Adolescents

Difficult as all this is for the normal teen-ager, the diabetic adolescent has the additional problems imposed by his disease. In the face of these new complexities, the care of adolescent diabetes becomes much more difficult than childhood diabetes.

First of all, and this seems a frightening thing to most parents, there is a very steep rise in the need for insulin. Daily requirements of 80 to 100 units are common. Parents ought not be disturbed by this—it is perfectly normal within the diabetes framework. Later, as the adolescent becomes an adult, the need for insulin will usually decline.

It should not be hard to understand why adolescents need more insulin than children or adults. Two factors are involved—calories and hormones.

In adolescence, metabolic activity is greater than at any other time. Growth demands greater caloric intake. At seventeen, a boy needs about 4,000 calories daily, almost twice what he will need as an adult. Most of these calories are taken as carbohydrates— bread, potatoes, cereals and the like, as well as fruits, ice cream, cake, and puddings. This in itself brings a sharp rise in the need for insulin.

The adolescent will spill more sugar into the urine despite the increased insulin. This, too, is perfectly normal and, in view of the huge carbohydrate consumption, should not worry parents unduly, provided the adolescent is growing well and shows none of the other diabetes symptoms.

Hormones are the other major reasons for the adolescent's big insulin need. As endocrine activity rises with adolescence, more hormones are poured into the blood—pituitary growth hormone, thyroid hormone, adrenalin and others. These substances tend to inhibit the activity of insulin and therefore more is needed to make up for the reduced efficiency.

Girls sometimes have an additional problem imposed by the endocrine changes that come with puberty. Regardless of the over-all rise in insulin need, menstruation may make an even further demand. The adolescent girl diabetic may find that starting about two days before the onset of her period she will need a larger dose of insulin. This increased dose will have to be maintained until about the second day of her period, then it can usually be brought back to normal. This rise and fall of insulin need in conjunction with the menstrual cycle may continue until the menopause.

Emotional Problems of Diabetic Adolescents

The impact of social and emotional problems upon diabetes is greater in adolescence than at any other time of life. And the diabetes, in its turn, has an equally disturbing effect upon the social and emotional adjustments of the adolescent.

The adolescent is more fervid about his rights and independence than the child or adult. Parental interference is particularly resented, since it is a symbol of childhood that the adolescent strives to shatter.

As he attempts to assert himself, the adolescent diabetic often uses his diabetes as a weapon of rebellion against his parents. He may run away from home without taking his insulin equipment with him. He may be slipshod about taking insulin. There may be a sudden resistance to the testing of urine.

The urine tests are a special problem to adolescent girls during menstruation. They frequently refuse to take any tests during the period. Here the understanding of the parents and the intelligent explanations of the physician are vital. Urine tests are essential in the treatment of adolescent diabetes and must not be discontinued for any reason.

Another form of adolescent resistance is that of going on an overnight date and delaying the morning insulin injection until the return home.

One girl of sixteen, who lived in a rather unfortunate home environment and felt rejected by her mother, used her diabetes as a means of escaping from home. Whenever the situation became unbearable, she would stop taking her insulin injections and go into severe ketosis. Her next stop would be the hospital where the care, attention, and treatment would restore her sense of personal value.

She liked the hospital so much that as soon as she was up and about, she would offer to help the nurses and do other things to make herself useful. After a number of these hospitalizations she became a nurses' aid and came to the hospital to live.

Parents should recognize that rebellion is a normal stage of adolescence whether or not diabetes is involved. They should not become panicked and try to over-control the adolescent or impose rigid restrictions. Usually this will only intensify the resistance. In most cases, the best way to deal with the situation is with tolerance and understanding. The adolescent should be allowed to express his individuality with an absolute minimum of interference. If the parent-child relationship has been a good one in the past, the chances are that the stage of adolescent rebellion will come and go with little, if any, disturbance to treatment.

Adolescent Patient Must Treat Himself

It is very important for parents to understand that full responsibility for all phases of diabetes control *must* rest with the adolescent patient. This is equally true whether the diabetes stems from childhood or is newly acquired. The parents must yield *completely* all of the daily chores relating to the disease.

Unless this is done, the revolt may either take a more serious turn or the adolescent may fail to mature properly. He may become overly dependent and unable to face the problems of adulthood.

Where the parent is mistrustful of the child's ability

to handle the disease and tries to exercise control indirectly or secretly, the adolescent is bound to sense it and become infuriated.

A mother, fearful that her diabetic son might go into insulin shock without anyone close knowing what to do, told her son's closest friend that her boy was diabetic. Swearing the friend to secrecy, she asked him to look out for the signs of insulin reaction and give her son candy or sugar when they occurred.

The next time they were at a party, the diabetic seemed to act a little light-headed while he was dancing with a girl; and the friend rushed over with candy. The diabetic boy, even though he was in the initial stage of an insulin reaction, knew immediately that the friend had been told his secret. And he also knew that the one who betrayed him could only be the parent.

That marked the end of the friendship; and the diabetic, fearful of further betrayals from his parents, hid his friendships from them and became even more withdrawn and secretive.

Bad as this situation is with boys, it is infinitely worse where the diabetic is a girl. For the adolescent girl, intensely conscious of her competition with other girls for the attention of boys and possible husbands, diabetes seems a tremendous handicap which must be kept secret. For a parent to divulge this secret to a close friend—who can only be a close competitor as well—would be unforgivable.

Parents must realize that secrecy is important to many adolescent diabetics during a stage of their growing up. The most intelligent thing they can do, with the assistance of the physician, is to teach the adolescent the importance of letting someone in the circle of friends know about the diabetes.

The choice of who is to be told must be left to the diabetic, and the parents should respect this right. Many emotional and social problems are involved in this choice. The adolescent girl, for instance, might feel far more secure if a close friend did *not* know about her diabetes. Instead she might choose to confide in one she does not view as a near competitor.

Frequently, adolescents who acquire diabetes are far better able to cope with the situation than their parents.

One such case occurred recently when a seventeen-year-old girl appeared at a doctor's office. Accompanying her were her mother and a procession of aunts. The fact that the girl had diabetes had already been determined.

While the doctor was examining the girl as a means of working out a pattern of treatment, the mother had an emotional outburst.

"Why couldn't this happen to me instead of my daughter?" she demanded tragically.

Despite herself the girl winced. The other relatives, in whispers just loud enough for the girl to overhear, asked such questions as: What will happen to her? How long will she live? Will she be able to marry? Will she be able to have children?

Fortunately, the girl had been going to boarding school. The doctor therefore advised that the girl return to school and take up her regular life with the addition of the insulin, the tests, and other necessities of treatment.

The girl did just that and handled herself extremely well. Later she reported that while she was at school her diabetes was no problem at all. It was only during vacations and holidays, when she returned to the emotionally charged home environment, that she was made self-conscious about her ailment.

Another problem of adolescent diabetes arises from the normal decline of communication between the growing child and the parent. The adolescent leaves the home, goes to school and spends increasingly more time away from home as he seeks to form a living pattern of his own.

Ordinarily this results in considerable anxiety on the part of any parent, but where the child is diabetic the situation may be much more serious. At this stage the parent should never attempt to *force* trust and communication. About the only fruit force can bear is hostility. On the other hand, if the parent's relationship with the child has been based on acceptance and understanding rather than on strict control and rigid obedience, the decline in parent-child communication may never become serious enough to create a major problem.

For the teen-ager, most of the childhood infections are no longer a danger. Colds and accidents, on the other hand, are problems but not necessarily serious ones. They result in a temporary increase in the need for insulin, which may differ with each individual. Diabetic boys also have a greater tendency toward acne, which may become a social problem.

Since adolescent girls become increasingly sedentary while boys become more active, the possibility of accident is more likely among boys. Despite the risk of injury and insulin shock, the diabetic adolescent should be encouraged to participate in sports and other physical activities.

Parents should not try to have diabetic children excused from gymnasium and athletic events.

There are two important reasons for this. It is vital for the adolescent's morale and sense of social status to be allowed to engage in normal activities. Secondly, physical activity makes the insulin he takes more efficient.

All the adolescent must remember, to avoid the possibility of shock, is to eat a bar of chocolate or drink a coke before the game.

Diabetic children should be allowed to run, jump, play baseball, basketball, or hockey. It would be well for parents to note that in the grueling game of tennis, two of America's outstanding stars have been diabetic since childhood. They are Billy Talbert and Ham Richardson.

Along with sports, all other normal social activities should be encouraged. There is no reason why diabetic adolescents should be less able than non-diabetics to stay out late, stay with a friend overnight, or even take a weekend or a vacation away from home. All that is needed is proper provision for the insulin injections and urine tests. The syringe can be carried in a Steritube, avoiding the need for sterilization; the injections and the urine tests can be performed in the privacy of a washroom.

Altogether, in sports, social and other activities, diabetes should not be allowed to become a problem.

Questions That Disturb Diabetic Adolescents

As the diabetic adolescent grows older and faces approaching adulthood, new problems rise up to disturb him.

What kind of future will he have? Will he be able to marry? Will he be able to meet the responsibilities of adult life? What sort of profession or career could he look forward to? Will he have any problem completing his education? Will he find a satisfactory place in society?

Such problems are faced by all adolescents, diabetic or not. But there is a difference. For the diabetic the problems are intensified as he uses them, consciously or unconsciously, to dramatize himself and his situation.

Diabetic girls are specially prone to fear the future and anticipate all sorts of hardships and obstacles in the way of a normal life.

These fears are usually groundless or vastly exaggerated.

Diabetes *does not* interfere with a girl's normal physical development. Nor does it interfere with the menstrual cycle. Diabetes *will not* prevent her from fulfilling the responsibilities of marriage; it *will not* rule out motherhood.

The future awaiting the diabetic is generally no different from that of the non-diabetic. It depends upon the individual and his relationship to the world around him. Only in some jobs, which we will discuss shortly, will the diabetes make any difference at all.

Regardless of reassurances, a number of adolescents are bound by personality to be uncertain and insecure in face of the future. If they happen to be diabetic, the underlying insecurity is heightened.

This is generally reflected in relations with members of the opposite sex and is usually more frequent and intense among girls. Where the diabetic is fearful about being unequal, he will be timid and hesitant about dating and "going out." Certainly, he will be reluctant to let his date know about his diabetes.

"To tell or not to tell" is one of the thorniest problems affecting the adolescent diabetic.

No major issues are involved on a casual date and there is no need to divulge one's diabetes. But if the dating is more serious and may turn into courtship, then the problem looms increasingly large. Ultimately, the diabetes must be revealed. The question is: When?

The diabetic with a wholesome attitude toward the disease and with no feeling of inferiority will probably tell about it at the start of courtship.

Those who are less secure will wait—and be torn by a sense of guilt for not telling. Girls often do not tell until the engagement is an accomplished fact.

Advice is neither possible or practical. Each diabetic will do what his or her personality permits and can live with. The insecure diabetic will tell when the guilt over-balances the insecurity. The secure diabetic will tell as soon as it seems important.

There is one point about this that can validly be made. Where a courtship or engagement breaks up over diabetes, the overwhelming probability is that the relationship did not have a sound basis to start with. Where there is a good relationship, diabetes is not used as a *reason* for breaking it up. It is only used as an *excuse* to end an unsound relationship which probably would have broken up on some other pretext if the diabetes did not exist.

Diabetes is *not* a barrier to marriage. The percentage of marriages among diabetics is about the same as among non-diabetics. Some diabetics marry with ease; some have disappointing episodes, with the diabetes used as an excuse. But, eventually, they marry.

Parents of non-diabetics will often oppose the marriage of their child to a diabetic for "medical reasons." Not only are these "reasons" usually invalid, but where there is a genuine emotional attachment, this opposition will be unsuccessful. Where marriage is concerned, some parents may oppose the free choice of their children in any case and will seize upon the most obvious excuse to make their opposition seem valid.

With modern-day management of diabetes, there is every reason for the diabetic boy or girl to approach the possibility of marriage secure in the knowledge that he or she will be every bit as good a partner as the non-diabetic, physically, emotionally, socially, financially, and intellectually.

What Careers for the Diabetic?

As far as higher education is concerned, diabetes is no problem. It does not impair the intelligence and has no effect on the ability to learn.

There is no restriction upon diabetics in college or professional schools. They may become nurses, doctors, lawyers, engineers or nuclear physicists, business administrators or bookkeepers for that matter.

Military service *is* closed to diabetics. The diabetic boy *will not* be drafted into the armed forces and can therefore plan his education or career *without* worrying about the loss of several years to military conscription.

While practically all of the professions and most jobs will be open to him, the young diabetic planning his future should recognize that certain fields remain blocked. A number of civil-service jobs, teaching for instance, are often closed to diabetics. So are police, fire-department and other hazardous jobs. In each case, the diabetics should check with his local civil-service board to learn which jobs are open and which are closed. He should also avoid accepting any job which might create a hazard to him or to the public as a result of possible insulin shock.

Diabetics who require insulin usually will not be able to get jobs operating public conveyances such as taxis, buses, trains and the like. They will be unable to become locomotive engineers, pilots of commercial aircraft or ship's officers. The reason is the possibility of insulin shock which, at a critical moment, might endanger the passengers.

The young diabetic should not be surprised if certain companies refuse him a job for no apparent reason *although they may claim that diabetes is not a factor.*

Actually, a number of outworn and threadbare prejudices still cling to some big-company employment practices. These are carry-overs from the old days when diabetics survived on semi-starvation diets and were consequently weak and not fully productive.

The prejudices are gradually disappearing and are bound to vanish completely when companies learn that with modern treatment the diabetic who eats well is as productive as the non-diabetic. As for the belief that diabetics are harder hit by infections and more prone to prolonged absenteeism—the advent of antibiotics has made infections such as pneumonia no more hazardous to diabetics than to non-diabetics. With modern drugs, intelligent care and long-acting insulin, the diabetic is as good a job risk as anyone else.

There is a further factor which may make some companies reluctant to employ diabetics. This is the matter of pensions. A number of civil-service and other organizations which have pensions or employees' insurance plans feel that diabetics may retire earlier than non-diabetics and thus make a smaller contribution to the pension or insurance fund.

Apart from these restrictions—which are not as extensive as they appear and many of which are being eased—the young diabetic can look forward to entering practically any profession for which he is qualified or taking virtually any position in business or industry.

His diabetes will have no appreciable effect upon his ability to compete with other young men or women for an education and a career.

Nor should it have any effect upon the diabetic's ability to achieve a successful marriage, win a respected place in society, and create a fruitful and attractive future.

CHAPTER 13

The Diabetic Adult

One of the many mysteries of diabetes is the way in which it varies with the age at which it is acquired. Not only does susceptibility increase as we get older, but the type of diabetes is usually milder.

This does not necessarily mean that the nature of the diabetes changes as the patient ages. The child with severe juvenile diabetes will have juvenile diabetes for the rest of his life. But the diabetes acquired at thirty is generally less severe than the diabetes acquired at ten. Furthermore, the problems of the disease change as the diabetic proceeds through the unfolding stages of his life.

One important fact about diabetes that *does not* change must be emphasized. At no point in the diabetic's life, from childhood to old age, should properly managed diabetes be considered a bar to the treatment of any illness or injury by medication, radiation, or surgery.

Many people fear that the treatment of other ailments may aggravate existing diabetes or that diabetes may impede the treatment of the ailment. *This is not true.* Where the diabetes is properly cared for, the diabetic can undergo any operation or take any medication as well as the non-diabetic.

Only ACTH, cortisone and its derivatives, and certain diuretics may affect diabetes. But, even here, if a diabetic needs these drugs for the treatment of arthritis, asthma, or some skin ailment, he may take them without danger, provided their possible ill effects are canceled by an increase in the insulin dose.

Since adulthood embraces that vast segment of life spanning from adolescence through old age, the problems of diabetes undergo significant changes along the way. The young adult, aged twenty to forty, has problems which differ markedly from those of the middle-aged adult of forty to sixty. And the problems of the middle-aged adult are hardly the same as those of the elderly, aged sixty and up. For this reason, each of the three major stages of adult life must be considered alone in terms of its own special character.

THE YOUNG ADULT

Diabetes is almost three times more frequent among young adults than among youngsters and represents a sort of transitional stage between the severe diabetes of the young and the mild diabetes of later adulthood. The acute onset typical of childhood is not as common. Ketosis and insulin shock are less frequent. The disease is generally more stable, less difficult to manage and less dependent on insulin.

About one-third of the cases of diabetes among young adults are acute, showing all of the classical symptoms of juvenile diabetes. Usually, these are recognized easily and quickly.

Another third of the cases also show the classical symptoms, but these are not as extreme or as disturbing.

The remaining third of the cases do not have the obvious symptoms, are not readily recognized and are generally detected casually during a physical examination for insurance, employment, or army induction. Among women, diabetes may be detected during pregnancy, which requires regular analysis of the urine.

Oddly, and here is another interesting facet of diabetes, those cases which show the classical symptoms will usually require insulin for treatment. This represents about two-thirds of young adult diabetics. Of these, perhaps 25 to 30 percent may respond to Orinase or other oral drugs.

The remaining third—those cases which were more difficult to detect—can usually be managed with oral therapy or, if the patient is overweight, a return to and maintenance of normal weight.

Among obese young adults, a weight reduction which is maintained may sometimes seem tantamount to a cure. This should never be taken for granted because, as they get older, their supply of available natural insulin may be further reduced by stress and the aging process. Should this happen, the diabetes would flare up again.

Treatment for the young adult who requires insulin resembles that of the juvenile except that the doses are smaller, and a single injection is usually enough for the whole day. Only a small number of young adults require an extra dose of quick-acting insulin.

There are two reasons why the young adult needs less insulin than the adolescent. Since he has stopped growing, his caloric needs are less. Furthermore, his living pattern is more regular.

Even if he has an acute onset of the disease, the young adult need not necessarily be hospitalized but can often be treated without undue interruption of his normal routine. The proper dose of insulin can be worked out by the physician as he evaluates the patient's daily response.

While the frequency of shock and coma is reduced

in young adults, they do occur and must be treated in the usual way.

Oversleeping is one of the frequent causes of insulin reaction among young adults. After a hard week's work, those extra hours of sleep on Saturday or Sunday morning may look especially attractive. But should this cause a delay in breakfast, shock may result. The same is true of social drinking, an extra hole of golf, or anything else that might make him delay or miss a meal.

Unusual physical activity remains a danger. The normally sedentary man who digs up the garden on the weekend runs the risk of shock.

On the other hand, the man who does hard physical labor during the week and rests up over the weekend may run the risk of ketosis unless he increases his weekend insulin dose.

Where the young adult does not take insulin, but manages with either diet or oral drugs, the possibility of shock or coma is reduced almost to the vanishing point. This enables him to face changes in social life, physical activity, and general routine without any great difficulty.

Apart from these relatively minor physical problems, the diabetes presents no great threat. The social and emotional problems which loom so large to the adolescent are almost non-existent for the young adult. Only in three areas do diabetic young adults face what appear to be serious problems—insurability, employability, and parenthood.

Of these, the matter of parenthood is by far the more upsetting.

Should Diabetics Have Children?

The question "Should diabetics have children?" actually consists of three subsidiary questions. These are: Can a diabetic have children? Can parenthood be dangerous to the diabetic? Will the diabetic parent have diabetic children?

The first two questions are easily answered. Today's adult diabetics, as a result of modern treatment of the disease, are normally fertile and *can* have children.

Parenthood poses no risk to either parent where one or both are diabetic. There is no threat to life, no aggravation of the disease. Diabetes in the husband in no way affects the pregnancy of the wife. Diabetes in the wife requires a closer attention and more careful supervision during the pregnancy. Beyond that it should cause no appreciable disturbance either to the woman or the childbearing.

The third question—whether diabetic parents will produce diabetic children—is more complex and requires a closer look at some widely accepted beliefs.

Heredity *does* play a part in the susceptibility to diabetes. Where a parent is diabetic, there is a greater chance of a diabetes-prone child being produced.

Where both parents are diabetic, there is a considerable risk of producing a diabetic child. But even this risk, while sizable, may not be as great as statistical prediction would indicate.

Genetically, a predisposition to diabetes appears to be inherited as a Mendelian recessive characteristic. This should make it possible to predict the chances of diabetes in a child if the condition of the parents is known. In actual practice, the facts are not as clear as they appear in theory. About all that can safely be said is that diabetes occurs more often in families with an appreciable history of diabetes.

In view of all this, should diabetics have children?

Yes, where one of the parents is diabetic.

Where both parents are diabetic, there should be considerably more weighing of the pros and cons. But even in those cases it is impossible to be dogmatic. People who want children enough and can have them, often will have them regardless of statistical risks.

Insurance for the Diabetic

Apart from the problems of parenthood—and employability, which was discussed in the chapter on the adolescent diabetic—the young adult faces the intensely practical problem of insurability. This could be of considerable moment where the diabetic is concerned with protecting his family against accident, illness, or death.

Today's diabetic need have no great worry about insurance. Until the mid-1940's, insurance companies rejected all diabetic applicants for life insurance. This rejection was based in great part on the prejudices and attitudes that had developed in the pre-insulin era. In more recent years, dozens of companies have taken another look at diabetes in terms of modern treatment. As a result there has been a complete change in attitude.

The diabetic who wants life insurance today can obtain it from a number of companies. But, as with anyone suffering a chronic ailment, his premium will be higher.

Diabetics can also have accident, health, hospitalization, and disability insurance at no increased premium, *but only as members of a group insurance plan*. Individual insurance of this type will be extremely difficult, if not impossible, for diabetics to obtain at present.

Many diabetics may also find it useful to know that the Veteran's Administration has recognized diabetes acquired during military service as justification for a disability pension. This pension can be obtained even where the diabetes develops *after* the discharge from service—*but no later than within one year afterward*.

It should also be noted that in most states, diabetics who apply for a driver's license must present a letter from their physician stating that the public would not be endangered if the diabetic were permitted to drive. The physician's judgement is based on the patient's susceptibility to insulin reaction. Where reaction is relatively rare and quickly checked, the diabetic driver should present no risk.

Beyond the impact of these major factors of parenthood, employability and insurability, the non-medical problems of diabetes are probably less for the young adult than for anyone else. Diabetes seems less threatening to him than to the adolescent who fears what will happen when he has to face the world on his own; or to the middle-aged or elderly diabetic over whom the fear of death casts a lengthening shadow.

For the young adult, the fulfillment of work, a career, and the raising of a family provide positive goals and incentives possessed by none of the other groups. He is more concerned with problems of achievement than of ailment.

THE MIDDLE-AGED DIABETIC

Between the ages of forty and sixty, diabetes becomes vastly more frequent and considerably less severe than in earlier years.

In middle age, the incidence of diabetes is almost ten times greater than among young adults. It also becomes about twice as frequent among women as men.

The number of middle-aged diabetics who show the obvious symptoms of the disease amounts to about half of the cases—considerably less than among young adults where two out of three have the classical symptoms.

These are the acute cases, and, until the development of Orinase, practically all required insulin injections. Today, only about 50 percent still need insulin; the rest can do well on oral drugs.

The remaining diabetics, half of the middle-aged total, do not have the obvious symptoms and the disease is usually detected during an examination for something else. In this group, if the patient is obese, a weight-reduction and maintenance diet is usually sufficient to control the disease. Where the patient is not obese, insulin or oral drugs may be needed.

Of all middle-aged diabetics, about 25 percent require insulin for treatment. The remaining 75 percent can be managed with oral therapy or diet alone.

Since the need for insulin is usually a direct indication of the severity of diabetes, the middle-aged type is patently less severe than the younger forms. There is less ketosis, less coma, and fewer incidents of shock. But stress, illness, accident, or surgery may increase the severity of the ailment and cause a need for insulin where no such need existed before. Once the emergency is over, treatment can usually return to normal.

It is at this stage in life that the symptoms of aging begin to make themselves evident. The most common of these is arteriosclerosis—hardening of the arteries—which develops in the normal as well as the diabetic population. Other ailments related to age also appears—coronary artery disease, hypertension, and strokes.

These ailments arise as part of the process of growing old. They are not unique to diabetics. But, where diabetes exists, they tend to occur somewhat sooner. It is as though diabetes accelerates the aging of the circulatory system. For this reason weight control is of particular importance to the middle-aged diabetic. Overweight—even mild overweight—seems to be a serious contributory factor in diabetes as well as in circulatory ills: A U.S. Public Health Service study shows that overweight individuals, whether or not they have a family history of diabetes, are more than twice as likely to become diabetic as people of normal weight.

Since all this is a problem affecting the total population at this age, there is no special solution for the diabetic. A tremendous amount of research into the causes and possible prevention or cure of this group of ailments is currently being done. Sooner or later the answers will begin to take shape, and these will apply equally to the diabetics and the non-diabetics who cross the threshold into the middle years.

THE ELDERLY DIABETIC

Past the age of sixty there is a continued increase in the incidence of diabetes. It is three times as frequent as in middle age.

To balance this climb, there is a decline in the severity of the disease. It is relatively mild in regard to urinary sugar, fewer cases require insulin, more can be managed with oral drugs or dietary control. There is also less ketosis and fewer incidents of insulin shock.

The disease itself seems to pose fewer difficulties, but the aging process creates a new set of problems in relation to the disease. So, while the possibility of shock is more remote, the consequences may be far more severe. Arteries become more brittle with age, and shock may now cause serious organic damage as a result—a heart attack or a stroke.

The elderly person, diabetic or not, is more prone to accident than in his middle years; more susceptible to certain illnesses; more likely to require surgery.

Where diabetes does exist, it should not be a problem interfering with proper treatment. But the stress of the acute illness, the accident or the operation may cause a change in the diabetes necessitating an increase of insulin or some other compensation in treatment.

For the elderly diabetic, the complications arising from arteriosclerosis are also more frequent and more severe than for the non-diabetic. Injury and infection, which caused no special problems for the younger diabetic, now are hazardous because of the decrease in blood circulation. Especially vulnerable are the feet, where circulation is usually most sluggish.

Special Precautions for Elderly Diabetics

There are a number of things the diabetic can do to protect himself from these complications of aging.

First of all, he can help his circulatory system by keeping his weight at normal or slightly below. Probably the best weight at this age is 10 percent below what is considered normal.

Equally important, he must take the proper precautions to avoid injury and infection, especially to the feet. Here, the diabetic should exercise common sense and observe such injury-preventing rules as the following: He should avoid ill-fitting shoes. He should avoid socks that are too large, too small or wrinkled. They may cause blisters or other damage. He should not walk barefoot, thus avoiding splinters or other injuries. He should exercise extreme care cutting his toenails. He should not apply powerful antiseptics such as iodine to delicate tissues. He should not attempt to trim his own corns or bunions or use corn or bunion removers which may be caustic. He should avoid extremes of heat or cold. Hot footbaths or hotwater bottles, if too hot, can be as dangerous as frostbite. He should be especially aware of the importance of cleanliness and hygiene. Feet should be washed carefully, at least once each day. Socks should be changed at least as frequently. He should be careful in choosing his work or recreation, avoiding activities which may cause injury, especially to the feet. An upholsterer, who frequently stepped on tacks, suffered serious complications. So did a night watchman on a building project after his feet became soaked in mud, then chilled. Equally hazardous are tasks involving the movement of heavy objects which may strike the feet.

These are some of the more obvious precautions. They should suggest others, fitted to each diabetic's individual pattern of living. Most important of all, the elderly diabetic should never attempt to treat injury or infection on his own. This should be left strictly to the physician.

Close contact with the doctor is vital at every stage of diabetes and is particularly important for the elderly patient. In any situation of stress, injury, infection or even where the slightest doubt or worry arises, the physician should be contacted at once.

The emotional problems of the elderly diabetic are in no way different from those of the non-diabetic. They usually center about a growing feeling of isolation and loneliness, a greater concern with death. There are no capsule solutions for these problems, depending as they do upon individual needs in relation to individual environments.

Any activity or situation which involves the elderly person and gives him a sense of continuing purpose is usually helpful. Anything which tends to further his isolation or a sense of declining usefulness is harmful.

The woman who tells her aging mother that she need no longer strain her eyes knitting sweaters for the grandchildren may unwittingly be causing great harm by destroying her mother's sense of being needed.

Old or young, diabetics have the same problems as other people their age in addition to the problems which may be unique to the disease. Except where the diabetes creates distinctly special needs, they should be treated like any other human being. In this way the diabetic will be free to live, love, work and function to fullest capacity possible.

CHAPTER 14

Diabetes as a Special Problem for Women

Although diabetes spares neither of the sexes, it poses some special problems for the female.

For one thing, diabetes seems to have a particular affinity for women. Of the estimated 2,000,000 diabetics in the United States, about 1,250,000 are female. What is more, of every 100 women and girls alive today, more than four are due to become diabetic.

The precise reasons for this are not fully known, although it seems virtually certain that metabolic and endocrine factors relating to childbearing and menopause are involved. Mothers, as has already been shown, are more susceptible than non-mothers; and, after the age of forty-five, women become twice as susceptible as men.

The fact that diabetes prefers women is not the only characteristic making it a special problem for the wife and mother. Women must take greater care in managing the disease than men. This is true for physiological reasons as well as for reasons arising from the everyday demands imposed upon the woman who must make a home and raise a family.

Finally, there is that most uniquely feminine complication of all to add to the problems of diabetes— that of pregnancy.

Before the advent of insulin and modern treatment, fertility was extremely low and diabetic women were rarely able to achieve pregnancy. Today the situation is completely reversed. With proper treatment, the diabetic woman is as fertile as the normal woman and has an equally high probability of surviving the pregnancy. What is more, where the chances of successful pregnancy were about nil in the pre-insulin era, today they have risen to better than 80 percent and, as treatment improves, will go even higher.

Non-diabetic women suffer a 4 percent loss of infants between the sixth month of pregnancy and the second day after birth. With diabetic mothers, where treatment is on a high level, the loss is only 6 percent higher.

The problems of pregnancy as they affect the diabetes are not particularly complex but they do demand careful attention.

Regardless of previous treatment during pregnancy the diabetic will require both diet and either insulin or, where possible, Orinase. Other oral drugs have not proved as harmless to the fetus.

Morning sickness, which is common during the first three months of pregnancy, may carry a threat of acidosis or insulin reaction. While serious to the mother, this can be far more dangerous to the unborn child. As a measure of protection, the prospective mother must be sure to take adequate nourishment. Where she has any difficulty with food or anything else, she must notify her physician at once.

Where the woman takes insulin, pregnancy often sends the insulin requirements into unpredictable gyrations. The needed dose may rise as much as two or three times normal or it may drop sharply for no apparent reason. Because of these wild changes, regular urine and blood tests for sugar and acetone become extremely important.

The pregnant diabetic has a greater tendency to spill sugar into the urine. This is not as significant as in the non-pregnant diabetic, but should be watched. Far more important would be the presence of acetone, which must be corrected without delay.

The diabetic woman has a greater-than-normal tendency to retain water in her tissues during pregnancy. For this reason a low-salt diet is usually important.

Where the diabetes has been well-treated, childbirth is more nearly normal. Stress, family and economic background are important factors. The woman with a good home environment usually has an easier time. The woman whose diabetes is relatively recent has a better chance of successful pregnancy than the woman with diabetes of twenty years or more.

Until about ten years ago, there was a much higher rate of infant loss among diabetics before, during and soon after birth. There was a higher percentage of spontaneous abortions and miscarriages. A number of infants seemed to develop well until about four weeks *before* birth, then they died in the womb for reasons still unknown. Another difficulty arose from the fact that diabetes in the mother often made the child too large for an easy or successful delivery.

Today, as the result of careful teamwork on the part of the mother's physician who cares for the diabetes, the obstetrician who attends to the pregnancy and delivery, and the pediatrician who cares for the infant after birth, there has been a dramatic improvement in the number of successful pregnancies.

Earlier Delivery Helps Successful Pregnancy

One of the most important contributions is made by a somewhat different approach to delivery. Instead of waiting for the pregnancy to run its full course, the baby is delivered before it either grows too large or dies in the womb during the last weeks of gestation.

The best time for delivery is usually during the 36th or 37th week of pregnancy, about 3 to 4 weeks before the normal time of birth. The optimum moment, which would allow for the fullest development of the infant as well as the best chances for a successful delivery, is determined by the obstetrician usually in consultation with the mother's physician.

Normal labor may be induced earlier by certain drugs or other methods or the baby may be delivered by Caesarian section. However it is accomplished, the technique of planned premature delivery has made it possible for the vast majority of diabetic women to achieve successful pregnancies. Then, with the pediatrician standing by to take over at birth, even the borderline infant has a good chance of survival.

Although the improvement has been enormous, successful pregnancy still remains more of a challenge for the diabetic than for the non-diabetic woman. Among the things making motherhood more difficult for the diabetic is the earlier tendency toward arteriosclerosis and an accelerated aging of certain organs. From this standpoint, a diabetic woman in her twenties seems to have the same problems as a normal woman in her forties. The over-all loss of infants from all causes during pregnancy and shortly after birth is about the same in both cases.

In Boston, one group of doctors headed by Dr. Priscilla White has been giving pregnant diabetics huge doses of hormones in an effort to improve even further the possibility of successful pregnancy. This hormone treatment, unfortunately, has not succeeded in producing the hoped-for results in the hands of others.

Meanwhile other work is going on at an increasing pace and the situation shows constant improvement. At The Mount Sinai Hospital in New York, during a ten-year period ending late in 1962, 243 pregnant diabetics were cared for. Receiving the best of modern "team" treatment involving the physician, obstetrician, and pediatrician, they produced a better than 90 percent record of successful births.

We have indeed come a long way from the pre-insulin era when pregnancy for the diabetic was most often either impossible or fatal.

Other Special Problems of Diabetic Women

Pregnancy is only one of the physiological problems that may complicate the diabetes of women.

Some diabetic women may have premenstrual difficulty. If they require insulin there may be a rapid rise in the needed dose shortly before menstruation; a sharp drop during or immediately after the period.

The menopause, with all its dynamic stresses, causes further changes and problems. At this time of life the tendency toward obesity seems to increase in women to a greater degree than in men. Since overweight can seriously complicate the diabetes, it becomes more important for women to watch their calories.

Insulin atrophy, rare in adult men, is not uncommon among women. This is not as serious physically as it is cosmetically and psychologically. The woman whose arms and legs are pitted because of this complication will be understandably reluctant to wear bathing suits or sleeveless dresses. While no cure is yet possible for the atrophy, the woman suffering it can certainly find many dress styles to fit her needs. The problem of the bathing suit is not so easily solved.

From young adulthood on, fungus infections in the genital area are more common among women. These can cause serious itching and discomfort. Where they exist, they can be treated with special fungicides which the physician will prescribe. Special hygienic care can also help prevent them.

As the diabetic woman enters middle age she becomes more susceptible than the man to bladder, kidney, and other urinary infections. Once these were a serious problem. Today, with a wide range of antibiotics at the disposal of the physician, the infections are amenable to control.

Diabetes also seems to increase a woman's vulnerability to heart ailments. Ordinarily, the healthy woman is three times *less* likely than a man to suffer from heart disease. Diabetes wipes out this advantage and makes the woman equally assailable.

Considering all these physiological factors, it is quite clear that even if everything else were equal, diabetes poses a greater problem for women than men.

Everything else is *not* equal if the woman is also a wife, and even less equal if she is a mother.

The average man lives a fairly regular life. He rises at a given time, eats at given times, has about the same amount of activity each day at his job. The very fact of a regular job usually imposes a set of regular habits which can be very helpful in the control of diabetes.

The wife, especially if she is also a mother, has an irregular life. Household emergencies are always arising to complicate the management of her disease.

A child takes sick and has to be treated at once.

Perhaps the child is hurt at outdoor play, and the mother has to fetch him home just as she is starting a required meal.

Her husband calls up about a last-minute dinner guest, so she has to run out for some emergency shopping.

These and events like them occur almost daily to upset the regularity of a housewife's life.

If she is taking insulin and these irregularities make her delay a meal or engage in too much physical activity, she may suffer a reaction. Even the best-organized homemaker cannot anticipate and be ready for all emergencies of cleaning, cooking, shopping, and child-raising.

Where the diabetic is a young adult, these problems are much more significant. Not only is it more likely that she will require insulin, but she is also more likely to be in the flush of building a family—a situation fairly bristling with emergencies and potential hazards.

On the other hand, this is not the case where the diabetes is controlled by diet alone or where oral therapy can supplant the need for insulin injections. Under those conditions, the problems lose their significance, since the diabetic woman is enabled to function more flexibly in the changing situations of daily life.

Looking back over the full range of diabetes problems as they affect women, the changes wrought by insulin, the oral drugs, and the over-all improvement of treatment have opened a whole new world of possibilities.

Because of these advances, the woman with diabetes is almost every bit as able as her non-diabetic sister to meet the responsibilities, emergencies, and pleasures of being a wife, a mother and everything that womanhood implies.

PART FOUR

The Prospects

CHAPTER 15

From Today
to Tomorrow

Up until about a century ago mankind was afflicted by a widespread disease known as *The Fever*. This strange malady showed certain peculiar variations. Some victims passed it off with scarcely any disturbance in their daily living. Others died. Regardless of the variations, one symptom was always present—the rise in temperature that gave the disease its name.

Treatment of The Fever consisted of lowering the temperature to normal. This involved the use of drugs similar to aspirin, sweating, purging, bleeding, and other practices then in vogue. In a great many cases the treatment was successful and the patients recovered.

Today we know that there was no such disease as The Fever. It was a catch-all designation for a whole range of fever-producing infections all the way from a severe cold to malaria, meningitis, typhoid, and pneumonia. We also know that each of these ailments, although they all produce the common symptoms of fever, is caused by a different microbe. Each of these microbes, in turn, is treated with specific antibiotics or other agents; and, once the cause is removed, the fever and other disease symptoms will vanish.

Today's diabetes resembles The Fever of a century ago in many respects. It shows considerable variation, but in practically every case there is a common symptom—a tendency to abnormally high blood sugar.

169

Treatment does not strike at the cause of the particular variety of diabetes involved. Instead it seeks to check the major symptom by reducing the sugar levels of the blood and urine.

Perhaps a century from now physicians will look back at us, shake their heads with benign tolerance and say:

"What the physicians of the mid-Twentieth century called diabetes was really a whole range of ailments, each with a different set of causes but with one symptom in common—abnormally high blood sugar. Since they couldn't distinguish between the causes of the different ailments, they could neither prevent nor cure them. Instead they treated the common symptom, using various means to keep the blood and urine sugar under control."

Considering how little we actually do know about the causes of diabetes, we have made remarkable progress in controlling the symptoms of the disease ever since the isolation of insulin. We have also developed a clearer understanding of some of the variations that make one case of diabetes differ from another.

Oral Drugs Revitalize Diabetes Research

In the years between the introduction of insulin and the discovery of the oral drugs, there was a sluggishness in diabetes research as well as a rigidity in-thinking about this disease. To many, the problem was as good as solved since the ailment in most cases could be fairly well controlled by insulin injections and diet. Consequently, interest in continued research and in the expansion of understanding waned.

During this period it was believed that every diabetic had an absolute deficiency of insulin.

Then, when the first sulfonylurea was introduced and showed that sulfonyurea drugs might be effective for a large number of adult diabetics, the prevailing lethargy was abruptly swept aside. A whole new group of investigators in all parts of the world turned their attention to the question raised by the oral drugs.

It was obvious, for instance, that these drugs were not insulin and had no insulinlike activity. Yet, the reponse they produced in the patient was one that could only occur in the presence of active insulin. Therefore it seemed clear that many of these diabetic patients *did* have insulin. However, it was somehow deficient or inactivated in the disease state but could be stimulated into activity by the drug.

As a result, it became apparent that the rigidly held belief that diabetes was due to an absolute deficiency of insulin was false, at least as far as the patients responsive to oral drugs were concerned.

Current research has indicated that many adult-onset diabetics not only have insulin but that many of them may have an abnormally high secretion of this hormone in the early stages of the disease, before it becomes overt. This has led J. Vallence-Owen of England to advance the concept that the prediabetic individual is often obese because the higher insulin level acts to synthesize more fat. In other words, he is obese because he is becoming diabetic, rather than becoming diabetic because he is obese.

Since it has been shown that the oral agents will prove successful in half of the maturity-onset diabetics, some insulin production and activity must be present in these individuals. In those diabetics who must include almost all the juvenile-onset diabetics, there may well be an absolute lack of insulin. However, a few juvenile-onset individuals do respond to the oral drugs, indicating that here, too, there are exceptional cases where the disease is not due to a lack of insulin but, rather, to an alteration in its ability to function. But even in these cases, as with some adult diabetics, the disease usually progresses until there is a total breakdown of the insulin mechanism.

Already, it is quite clear that since the introduction of tolbutamide, a revolution has taken place in diabetes classification, thinking, and research. The diabetes can now be further refined to include those forms of diabetes in which insulin is present and those in which it is absent.

With diabetes found to exist even in patients who had pancreatic insulin, investigators turned their attention to the possible factors that could produce such an apparent contradiction. This has led to the discovery of insulin binding; insulin antibodies; insulin antagonists in the albumin fraction of the blood proteins; and abnormal insulin which, because of a possible enzyme defect, cannot perform its metabolic function.

Another defect that has been found is one of timing in the release of insulin by the pancreas. Where this exists, in both juvenile and adult diabetics, the pancreas produces insulin in an amount sometimes even larger than normal. But the release of this insulin is somewhat delayed so that it does not synchronize with the rise in blood sugar that follows a meal. This causes a failure in carbohydrate metabolism.

So, in addition to helping achieve a more precise classification of diabetes and the delineation of several previously unsuspected varieties of the disease, the advent of the oral drugs has directed research to a number of defects in the insulin mechanism which may cause diabetes. This, in turn, opens the way to investigations which may lead to possible means of preventing the development of these defects in those who are susceptible and in correcting them where they do occur.

Diabetes and Glandular Disturbances

Although glandular disturbances other than those of the pancreas have been implicated in some cases of diabetes, it should be understood that these play a very limited role. Actually, less than one case of human diabetes in a thousand can be attributed to such a cause. Yet they do exist and should be given some consideration, but no more than is indicated by their limited importance.

At the Mayo Clinic in Rochester, Minnesota, there was a patient who had been suffering from diabetes for five years and required large doses of insulin. This diabetic also had a tumor of the adrenal gland which is located atop the kidneys. The tumor was removed by surgery and, as soon as it was gone, the diabetes symptoms vanished. The patient no longer required insulin and had a normal sugar tolerance thereafter.

Overactivity of the thyroid gland, which seems to speed up the metabolic needs of the patient, may also be accompanied by diabetes symptoms in about 20 to 30 percent of the cases. In a number of these, where the hyperthyroid condition was corrected by surgery, radioactive iodine, or drugs the symptoms of diabetes disappeared. In some cases they later returned, in other cases the remission seemed permanent.

A tumor of the anterior pituitary gland which causes acromegaly—an enlargement of the face, hands, and feet—is associated with diabetes symptoms in about 20 to 30 percent of the cases. Where the pituitary gland is destroyed, the diabetes will disappear.

The disease known as Cushing's Syndrome, which may result from tumors of either the pituitary or adrenal gland, in almost every case is also accompanied by the symptoms of diabetes. Wherever there is a successful cure of the tumor, the diabetes also seems to vanish.

A study made by J. P. Kriss and P. H. Futcher showed that 77.1 percent of the women who gave birth to a child weighting ten pounds or more developed diabetes within an average period of 24.2 years after the child's birth. Mothers who had babies weighing thirteen pounds or more all developed diabetes in time. Since the size of the child is related to the mother's production of pituitary growth hormone, scientists suspect that this hormone may be involved in a form of diabetes.

An even closer correlation between large infants and maternal diabetes was seen in a U.S. Public Health Service study by J. B. O'Sullivan in 1961. This showed that among women who gave birth to large infants of nine or more pounds and who had a transiently abnormal glucose tolerance test, 28.5 percent became diabetic after five and a half years. Also included in this high-risk category were women who had obstetric difficulties such as spontaneous abortion, miscarriage, or toxemia of pregnancy.

This relationship was further supported by an experiment conducted by F. G. Young in England. Young gave pituitary growth hormone to puppies and kittens. All it did was stimulate further growth while they were still growing. But after they stopped growing, administration of the hormone produced diabetes.

Certain drugs seem to produce the symptoms of diabetes. These include ACTH, cortisone, prednisone, and similar substances which are actually duplicates of hormones made by the pituitary and adrenal glands. While very useful in arthritis and other ailments, in a small percentage of cases these drugs seem to provoke what is known as steroid diabetes. This can be very severe but has been known to disappear when the drugs are discontinued. In other cases, where the drug seems to make latent diabetes flare up, the disease will remain. Since physicians are now alert to the situation, they watch patients for signs of diabetes while administering any of these drugs.

In all these cases, the diabetes seems to result from some imbalance or malfunction of the endocrine system, or the excessive presence of some hormone.

But the way in which the disease symptoms are produced is not necessarily the same.

An overactive thyroid, by speeding up metabolism and making great demands on insulin, may produce diabetes by creating a relative insufficiency of insulin.

Excessive growth hormone may produce diabetes symptoms by inhibiting the activity of insulin.

Diabetes symptoms are also induced by situations not directly related to the glands and hormones. There are many factors in the blood and cell tissues which may inhibit the proper metabolism of carbohydrates.

In the blood, insulin may be bound, blocked, or destroyed by certain antagonists and antibodies which ordinarily are formed to fight disease-producing organisms. S. A. Berson and R. S. Yalow, working in New York, have shown that antibodies against insulin can produce experimental diabetes in animals. They have also found such antibodies circulating in the blood of individuals who need huge doses of insulin to control their diabetes. This form of insulin resistance is evidently due to the presence of high blood levels of insulin antibody, which may also play a possible role in causing diabetes in some patients.

Another possible factor in producing diabetes may be abnormalities in the form of the insulin available to the body. Recent investigations by H. Antoniades in the United States reveal that free insulin released by the pancreas may, when it reaches the liver, be joined to a protein which inactivates it. He found that in normal people there is a rise in free insulin in the blood following a meal, while the protein-bound to the albumin in the blood, itself becomes a rise mainly of the protein-bound, or inactive, insulin.

An additional blood protein, albumin, may also be involved in insulin antagonism. The insulin molecule, it is now known, is made of two parts linked together, the A-chain and the B-chain. J. Vallence-Owen has noted that the B-chain, when bound to the albumin in the blood, itself becomes an antagonist to insulin activity. This substance, known as *synalbumin*, may be another element in the process of diabetes development in man.

The insulin elaborated in the pancreas may also be of an abnormal type, one with sufficient variation in chemical structure to make it incapable of serving its metabolic function.

Insulin may be prevented from penetrating into to cells and tissues where it is needed. In other cases, it may be destroyed in the tissues by certain substances such as the enzyme *insulinase.* This enzyme is present in all people, non-diabetic as well as diabetic, and is made principally in the liver as well as in some other tissues. However, its possible role in the production of diabetes is not clear.

Faced with a variety of differing possibilities—any one of which may set into motion the conditions leading to diabetes—it becomes extremely difficult for doctors to make a specific diagnosis. They cannot, for instance, tell a patient that he is suffering from a disorder of the pituitary gland which is reducing his ability to utilize sugars.

About all they can say is that the patient has diabetes and, since they do not know the specific mechanism causing the disease, they cannot prescribe a specific treatment or cure. Instead, they must use the present method of treatment—that of keeping the symptoms under control.

There is only one variety of diabetes about which the cause is clearly known. That is where the pancreas is removed by surgery or destroyed by disease and no source of native insulin remains. In these cases, the injection of insulin is the specific treatment.

Remissions and the Possibility of Cure

Diabetes, at present, is considered an incurable disease. This does not mean that it will always be so or that every case of existing diabetes cannot be cured. Some cases, like the one in which the removal of a tumor from the adrenal gland ended the diabetes, are cured.

Actually, when medicine talks about effecting a cure it means something more than the mere disappearance of symptoms. *Predictable cause and effect are also involved.*

If a person has a disease which vanishes for some unknown reason, that cannot be considered a cure. It is known as a spontaneous remission of symptoms.

A cure can be claimed only when a person who has a disease is given a certain treatment and, as a direct result of that treatment, the symptoms vanish and the patient returns to normal. What is more, the action of the treatment should be predictable and work the same way against the same disease every time. In this way penicillin is a cure for pneumonia because it will destroy the microbe that causes pneumonia with statistical certainty.

The diabetes "cures" that have occurred are more in the nature of remissions. Permanent remissions do happen, although they are rare. More frequent are the temporary remissions. In just about every case, the exact mechanism behind the remission is unknown. Sometimes a remission may even contradict an accepted cause-and-effect principle.

For instance, a United States Army lieutenant developed an unusually severe diabetes and was so insulin-resistant that he needed 270 units a day— an exceptionally large dose. Then, all at once, his diabetes seemed to vanish. For five years, he was absolutely free of any symptoms, living a perfectly normal life when, as mysteriously as it had disappeared, the diabetes returned.

Remissions also take place in juvenile diabetes after insulin treatment is begun. But the disease invariably returns. However, it may be possible today to prolong this remission for months or even a year or more by the use of oral drugs. But even in these cases the diabetes must be expected to return.

In many cases of mild diabetes, the simple dietary measures of avoiding concentrated sugars and reducing calories are often enough to eliminate abnormal blood sugar and other symptoms permanently or for many years. In other apparently identical cases, the ailment may suddenly flare in severity.

Even in some cases of flagrant diabetes—where the symptoms are not at all mild—simple dietary measures may bring a total disappearance of the disease, which is maintained as the years go by.

Then, as we discussed in an earlier chapter, illness, pregnancy or stress—emotional as well as physical—may provoke the symptoms of diabetes for a brief period, after which they vanish only to return again at some future time.

In all of these situations, the apparent "cure"—be it temporary or permanent—can hardly be claimed as a predictable result of some specific treatment as is the case with pneumonia when penicillin is used. It is for this reason that diabetes, despite the possibility of remissions, is considered incurable. It will only become curable when we are able to predict the remissions, control them, and make them permanent.

Can Diabetes Be Prevented?

There is another area of research which promises to produce useful results. This is the possibility of predicting who is likely to develop diabetes and then, by prophylactic treatment, preventing it.

In some cases, the question "Who is pre-diabetic?" can already be answered: The mother of oversized children may be pre-diabetic. The mother of many children may be pre-diabetic. The person with a considerable family history of diabetes may be pre-diabetic.

In addition to these clues there are several tests which may indicate a predisposition to diabetes. None of these should be considered absolutely accurate or final in any way. All we can say is that they appear to open possible avenues of approach to the problem.

The first test deserving of mention is the sugar tolerance test which is often used as a means of detecting diabetes where no apparent symptoms exist. In this test, the subject is given an abnormally large amount of sugar, and if he cannot handle it, diabetes is considered present.

Ordinarily, a person who has a normal response to a sugar-tolerance test is diagnosed as non-diabetic. Now, let us assume we are testing a person with a family history of diabetes. The results are negative and he has no diabetes. Then we take the test a step further.

An hour before the sugar-tolerance test he is given cortisone or an injection of ACTH which sometimes tends to block normal insulin activity. Following this his response to the test may be abnormal. This does not mean that he has diabetes. But it may, under certain circumstances, be considered a sign that he is due to become diabetic some time in the future.

The concept of detecting potential diabetic individuals stems from the very careful work of J. W. Conn and S. S. Fajans at the University of Michigan. These investigators followed a large number of children and young adults who showed this minimal abnormality, and they have been able to prevent its progression to overt diabetes by the prolonged administration of small doses of Orinase.

This still-experimental preventive procedure has been more successful in younger than in older individuals showing a similar minimal metabolic defect. This would suggest that possible diabetes prevention might find its likeliest candidates among children, adolescents, and young adults.

The first step in this type of program, obviously, would be the refinement of such tests as the cortisone-glucose tolerance determination. Applying such a screening technique to individuals with a family history of diabetes, or with some abnormality or sign suggestive of the potential development of diabetes, the pre-diabetics might then be identified and steps taken to prevent the onset of the disease.

That such a possibility may be well within reach was indicated by Conn and Fajans when they summarized their results as follows:

"Carbohydrate tolerance improved or became normal in seventeen of twenty young, monobese, mildly diabetic patients after prolonged treatment with tolbutamide. The improvement has persisted for as long as four years.

"The results suggest that prolonged administration of tolbutamide to such patients actually improves performance of the insulin-producing tissue in addition to the acute action of this compound in facilitating release of insulin.

"These studies suggest the possibility that beta cell decompensation might be preventable if administration of sulfonylurea compounds is initiated before carbohydrate tolerance is lost."

Since diabetes undoubtedly involves a number of different disease mechanisms, it is hardly likely that one test will suffice for all pre-diabetic conditions. Nevertheless, if these tests only help distinguish between one form of diabetes and another, they will be giving a considerable boost to our knowledge.

At present, two definite steps might be taken in an effort to prevent the development of diabetes. One of these is the correction of obesity. The second is the prophylactic use of sulfonylurea drugs where strong suspicion of impending diabetes exists.

Basic Research Providing Vital Clues

A great advance in our understanding of insulin was made when F. Sanger of Cambridge, England, successfully accomplished the monumentally difficult task of breaking down the complex insulin molecule and showing its structure. As a result, scientists were enabled to know the essential components of the molecule and how they are linked together. This knowledge led to the successful synthesis of insulin by P. G. Katsoyannis in Pittsburgh in 1963.

When Sanger unlocked the insulin molecule and showed its structure, it was seen that the hormone was built of two pairs of chemical chains—two A-chains and two B-chains forming a complete arrangement.

The A- and B-chains, it was then postulated, may be two opposing substances; the A-chain having insulin activity as we know it, the B-chain acting as an antagonist to block this activity or damp its effect, thus serving as a regulator. Apparently, through the process of natural selection, this molecule has so evolved that it can normally maintain a balance between insulin need and the hazard of insulin excess which might result in hypoglycemia.

Today, it has become possible to anticipate the creation of a synthetic insulin that would be effective if taken orally. This might be based on active A-chain or even part of the chain and, by virtue of smaller molecular size and weight, might be able to pass through the digestive tract unchanged.

Such an oral insulin would eliminate the secondary problems created by the need to inject insulin. It would be absorbed along with the food and passed directly into the liver, the strategic point where natural insulin and absorbed food ordinarily come together.

Should this possibility be realized, the diabetic patient could expect great benefit as regards treatment.

A more immediate research prospect is the creation of insulin molecules with radioactive tags. These will enable scientists to trace the path of the hormone through the body and thus determine its metabolic pathways and fate. This is bound to lead to a fuller understanding of where and how insulin works and how some forms of diabetes may be caused.

Meanwhile, newer drugs with which to treat diabetes continue to be sought. Spurred by the success of Orinase, Diabinese, Dymelor, and DBI, researchers are striving to discover other compounds which might do an even better job.

The United States Government, at the National Institutes of Health in Bethesda, Maryland, is conducting a crash program in which it is screening many chemicals, natural and synthetic, for possible antidiabetic effects. A number of the pharmaceutical companies have similar programs under way.

In another area of research currently being explored, it has been found that certain changes take place in the body, apparently in advance of the onset of clinical diabetes. These tissue changes, which may be premonitory of blood sugar abnormalities, have aroused deep interest in many research centers throughout the world.

At Joslin Clinic in Boston, investigators have detected changes in the elastic tissue of the ear lobes of diabetes-prone individuals on the verge of acquiring the disease. Similarly, changes have been found in certain blood constituents other than sugar; in the diameter of blood vessels which can be seen at the surface of the eye; and in the connective tissue of the basement membrane of the kidney. Changes have also been measured in the nature of pulsations of the arteries in the extremities.

Much of the original work in this area was done by J. Ditzel and R. Camarini-Davalos at Joslin Clinic. It seemed so promising that other scientists soon took up the study of possible pre-diabetic tissue changes.

Since these alterations are presumed to be preliminary to the onset of clinical diabetes, Camarini-Davalos administered prophylactic doses of tolbutamide to probable pre-diabetics who showed some of these advance tissue changes but had no blood sugar abnormalities. He found that his treatment arrested the otherwise progressive nature of the changes which, untreated, would have continued to develop until full-blown clinical diabetes became manifest.

This work is continuing and, along with that of Conn and Fajans, offers great promise of possible prevention of diabetes in the not too distant future.

Altogether, the research prospects look good.

For thousands of years our knowledge of diabetes was frozen by ignorance and the prejudice it engendered. Today there is vigorous activity on a world scale. All aspects of diabetes are involved in the research, from basic causes to new forms of treatment. True, the work is scattered and uncoordinated—all of which undoubtedly causes a drag. But the progress is there and it will inevitably gain momentum as more is discovered. Then, in some not-too-distant tomorrow, the causes and possible cures will come into clearer view.

For the present, although we have not yet mastered diabetes, we have learned to control it. It is no longer almost invariably fatal. We can detect it, treat it, curb its symptoms, reduce its complications and cope with most of its problems. What is more, we can do these things with a minimum of intrusion into the ordinary routines of daily living.

As a result, whatever promises are still to be fulfilled by the expanding future, today's diabetic can live a longer, fuller and more nearly normal life than was ever before imagined possible.

Index

Abel, J., 66
Aborption (spontaneous), 174
Acetest, 80, 89
Acetohexamide, 97, 103
Acetone, *see* Ketone
A-chain, 175, 181
Acidosis, 20, 69, 84, 98, 113, 114, 125, 130, 157
Acne, 144
ACTH, 17, 113, 150, 174, 179
Addison's disease, 95
Adolescence, 22, 30, 31, 110
Adolescent diabetes, 138-149
Adolescent rebellion, 138, 140-141
Adrenal gland, 173
Adrenalin, 139
Adult diabetes, 31-33, 35, 59, 71, 93, 95, 149-159
Alcohol, 51, 59, 108, 109
Allen, F. M., 41, 56, 57, 62
Allen diet, 41, 56, 57
Allergy, 76
Alpha cells, 17
American Diabetes Assn., 59, 78, 81

American Dietetic Assn., 59
Ames Co., Inc., 88, 89
Anabolism, 19
Antibiotics, 46, 94, 105, 148, 165, 169
Anticipation factor, 26
Antihistamines, 76
Antoniades, H., 175
Aretaeus of Cappadocia, 39
Arteriosclerosis, 118, 156, 157, 163
Arthritis, 150, 174
Asthma, 150
Athletics and sports, 144
Augusta-Viktoria Hospital, 93

Baker Clinic, 55
Banting, F. G., 16, 57, 62, 65
Barmbeck General Hospital, 93
Barron, M., 62, 63
B-chain, 175, 181
Beckton, Dickenson & Co., 78
Bedford Survey, 22
Bedwetting, 33, 128
Benedict solution, 88
Berson, S. A., 175
Bertram, F., 93

185

Best, C. H., 16, 57, 64-65
Blood-sugar, 31, 43, 69, 83, 91, 93, 107, 108, 126, 169, 170
Bouchardat, A., 51
Bran, 57
Brittle diabetes, *see* Juvenile diabetes
Burroughs, Wellcome & Co., 77
BZ-55, 93, 94

Caesarian section, 163
Calories, 24, 31, 53, 56, 59, 138, 151
Camarini-Davalos, R., 182
Camps for diabetic children, 131, 136
Candy, 34, 41, 110, 111, 116, 126
Cantani, A., 51
Cantani Diet, 51
Carbohydrates, 13, 14, 20, 31, 32, 34, 38, 41, 42, 43, 50, 51, 53, 55, 56, 59, 84, 91, 112, 132, 133, 139
Careers and jobs, 105, 144, 147, 148, 155
Catabolism, 19
Cawley, T., 14, 15
Cézanne, P., 37
Chicken pox, 31
Childbearing, 23, 160
Childhood diabetes, 123-137
Children, 22, 30
Chlorpropamide, 97, 103
Circulatory system, 18, 36, 156, 158
Clemenceau, 37
Clinistix, 80, 88, 89
Clinitest, 80, 88, 89
Collip, J. B., 65
Coma, *see* Diabetic coma
Complications, 89, 101, 106-120, 157, 158
Conn, J. W., 179, 183
Cortisone, 17, 150, 174, 179
Cortisone-Glucose Tolerance Test, 179
Crystalline insulin, 66
Crystalline zinc insulin, 66-69, 72
Cushing's syndrome, 173

Dating, 146
DBI, 46, 97, 100, 103, 182
Denver Chemical Co., 89
Diabetes *(diabetes mellitus)*, 13, 28, 33; possible causes, 16-28, 170-177, 183; possible cure, 176-179, 183
Diabetes classification, 170-172
Diabetes prevention, 178-180, 183
Diabetes research, 170, 172, 180-183
Diabetes susceptibility, age factor, 21, 22; sex factor, 22, 23; heredity factor, 24
Diabetic coma, 34, 55, 69, 73, 106, 112, 119
Diabinese, 46, 97, 100, 101, 103, 182
Diagnosis, 18, 19, 24
Diet, 25, 32, 40, 41, 49-61, 157, 170
Diuretics, 113, 150
Dixon, G. H., 46
Dogs, 15, 61, 63-64
Dosage, DBI, 100-103; Dymelor, 100, 103; Insulin, 30, 31, 37, 65, 66, 67, 72, 78, 81, 82, 84, 87, 99, 100, 108, 113-118, 128, 131, 135, 139, 140, 152, 160, 161; Orinase, 95, 100, 103

Driver's license, 154
Du, Y. C., 46
Ductless glands, *see* Endocrine glands
Dymelor, 100, 103

Eaton, J. C., 23
Ebers, G., 38
Ebers Papyrus, 14, 38
Education, 131, 147
Emotional problems, 34, 123, 124, 125, 134, 138, 152
Employability, 105
Endocrine glands, 27, 38, 138, 139
Energy, 19, 37, 51, 60, 113, 117, 138
Enzymes, 172, 176

Fajans, S. S., 179, 183
Farbwerke Hoechst Co., 94
Fasting, 52, 54, 56, 57, 70
Fat atrophy, 89, 164, 165
Fatigue, 29
Fats, 20, 24, 50, 51, 55, 56, 117
Feet, 157, 158
"Fever," 169
Folin, O., 61
Food & Drug Administration, 96, 98
Frank, E., 91
Franke, H., 93
Fuchs, K. J., 93
Fungus infections, 164
Futcher, P. H., 173
Gallstones, 63
Geography as diabetes factor, 24, 25
Gilchrist, J., 16, 64, 66, 69
Glasgow Diabetes Clinic, 23
Glen, A., 23
Globin, 68, 69
Globin zinc insulin, 68, 74, 84

Glucagon, 17, 80, 111
Growth, 34, 44, 60, 128, 139
Growth hormone, 17, 27, 139, 174, 175
Guelpa, Dr., 53, 54
Guelpa treatment, 53, 54

Hagedorn, H. C., 67
Hallas-Møller, 68
Harvard University, 61
Heart disease, 156, 157, 165
Heredity, 26, 27, 153, 178, 179
Hunger, 29, 33
Hygiene, 18, 158, 164
Hyperthyroidism, 58, 171
Hypodermic syringe, 68, 78, 79, 86
Hypoglycemia, 85, 102, 107
Ice cream, 133, 134, 135
Identification cards, 80, 109
Indians, 25
Infections, 27, 29, 36, 89, 104, 125, 135, 157, 159, 169
Insulin, 16, 18, 26, 30, 32, 38, 42, 46, 57, 59, 89, 90, 97, 105, 131, 132, 135, 152, 153, 154-158, 166, 170-173, 176, 177-181; allergy, 76, 77, 99, 105; antagonists, 172, 175, 180, 181; atrophy, *see* Fat atrophy; binding, 172, 175, 176; deficiency, 26; injections, 34, 42, 81-83, 126-131; mixtures, 68; oral, 181; reaction or shock, 34, 45, 60, 68, 85, 104, 105, 106-113, 128, 148; resistance, 177; storage and temperature, 77, 86; types (chart), 76

Insulinase, 17, 176
Insulin-deficient diabetes, *see* Juvenile diabetes
Insulin synthesis, 181
Insurance for diabetics, 154
Islets of Langerhans, 16, 62, 63, 65, 92, 98, 105
Israel, 25
Itching, 29, 36, 164

Janbon, M., 92
Jobs, *see* Careers
Johns Hopkins University, 62, 66
Joslin, E. P., 49, 57
Joslin Camp, 58
Joslin Clinic, 182
Juvenile diabetes, 27, 30-32, 33, 35, 68, 71, 73, 93, 95, 138, 149, 150

Katsoyannis, P. G., 46, 181
Ketone (acetone), 20, 55, 86, 113
Ketosis, 34, 113-117
Ketostix, 80, 89
Kidneys, 18, 29, 36, 91, 105, 165
Kleiner, I. S., 62
Kriss, J. P., 173
Külz, R. E., 53

LaGuardia, F. H., 37
Lancereaux, E., 14
Langerhans, P., 15
Lente insulin, 68, 75, 76, 114
Lilly & Co., Eli, 76, 80, 81, 88, 94, 97
Liver, 17, 27, 38, 91, 105, 175
Loubotières, A., 92

MacGregor Instrument Co., 78

MacLeod, J. J. R., 63
Malaria, 169
Marriage, 145, 147, 149
Maturity-onset diabetes, *see* Adult diabetes
Mayo Clinic, 173
Meal schedules, 83, 84, 90, 104, 126, 131, 135, 165
Measles, 31
Meningitis, 169
Menopause, 22, 23, 160, 164
Menstruation, 140, 145
Merck, Sharp & Dohme, 77
Meredith, Capt., 49, 50
"Metabolic Sundays," 52
Metabolism, 13, 16, 18, 19, 20, 25, 38, 43, 55, 91, 115, 172, 175, 181
Metropolitan Life Insurance Co., 55
Microbes, 169
Military service and conscription, 147, 154
Milk diet, 52
Minkowski, O., 62, 63
Miscarriage, 174
Montpellier Clinic, 92
Montpellier, University of, 92
Morning sickness, 161
Motherhood, 147
Mount Sinai Hospital, 96, 163
Munro, H. N., 23
Murlin, J. R., 62

Natal, 25
National Institutes of Health, 182
National Research Council, 58
Nationality, 24, 25
Naunyn, B., 15, 52, 55
Nausea, 102

NPH (Neutral Protamine Hagedorn) insulin, 68, 74, 75, 84, 114

Oatmeal diet, 52

Obesity, 19, 23, 30, 32, 59, 156, 164

Obstetrician, 162-164

O'Donovan, C. J., 95, 96

Opie, 62

Oral drugs, 34, 45, 46, 59, 90, 98, 99, 106, 151, 152, 156, 157, 161, 166, 170-172, 181; types (chart), 103

Orinase, 32, 45, 46, 60, 71, 90, 95-103, 151, 155, 161, 182

O'Sullivan, J. B., 174

Overeating, 25, 32

Overweight, see Obesity

Pancreas, 14, 15, 16, 32, 33, 38, 42, 62, 65, 97, 105, 175, 176

Paracelsus, see Von Hohenheim

Parenthood, 152, 153

Pediatricians, 44, 162-164

Pfizer & Co., Chas., 81, 97

Phenformin, 97, 103

Physical activity, 85, 86, 114, 130, 132, 152

Piorry, P. A., 41

Pituitary gland, 17, 27, 138, 139, 173, 174; Pituitary growth hormone, see Growth hormone

Pneumonia, 115, 169, 178

Pre-diabetes, 169, 171; early signs, 182; tests, 178, 180; tissue changes, 182

Prednisone, 174, 178, 179

Pregnancy, 23, 29, 151, 153, 160-164, 174, 178

Premature delivery, 163

Professions, see Careers

Protamine, 67, 68, 69

Protamine zinc insulin, 67-69, 73, 84, 114

Proteins, 17, 19, 24, 41, 50, 55, 56, 59

Puccini, G., 37

Race, 24, 25

Rastinon, see Orinase

Research, see Diabetes research

Regular insulin, 66-69, 72, 132

Remissions, 36, 127, 176-178

Richardson, H., 144

Rockefeller Institute, 56

Rollo, J., 41, 49

Rollo diet, 41, 50, 51

Sanger, F., 180

Scurvy, 38

Secrecy concerning diabetes, 109, 142-143

Semilente insulin, 76

Sharpey-Schafer, Sir E., 62

Shock, see Insulin shock

Skin disorders, 29

Social drinking, 109, 152

Squibb & Sons, E. R., 77, 81

Starch, 13, 16, 17

Starvation, 19, 20, 57, 61

Sterilization of equipment 79, 82, 86

Steritube, 79, 82, 86, 145

Steroid diabetes, 174

Stillbirth, 36

Stress, 27, 29, 33, 104, 116, 118, 151, 178

Sugar, 13-16, 20, 25, 60, 107-115, 116, 117

Sugar substitutes, 111

Sugar tolerance test, 179
Sulfa drugs, 92, 93, 94, 103, 105
Sulfonylurea, 94, 97, 100, 103, 105
Surgery, 98, 104, 149, 156
Sweet drinks, 110, 111, 116, 117, 131
Symptoms, diabetes and diabetic coma, 29, 33, 35, 36, 112-113, 117, 150, 155, 156; insulin reaction and shock, 109-112, 117
Synalbumin, 176
Synthalin, 91, 94

Talbert, B., 37, 144
Talcum powder, 57
Tes-tape, 80, 88
Thirst, 29, 33, 35
Thyroid gland, 17, 27, 173, 175
Tolbutomide, see Orinase
Tolinase, 97, 100, 101, 102, 103
Tolstoi, E., 119
Travel, vacations, 86, 145, 177
Tumors, 173, 174, 177
Typhoid, 92, 169

Ultralente insulin, 75, 76
Unit of insulin, 66, 72, 77
University of Toronto, 63
Upjohn Co., 81, 94-96
Urinary infection, 177
Urinary sugar, 14, 41, 42, 104, 116, 120, 126, 130, 157, 170

Urination, 29, 35, 36, 130-132
Urine tests, acetone, 72, 80, 86, 88, 116, 128, 141, 161; sugar, 71, 80, 86, 88, 116, 117, 141, 161
U. S. Public Health Service, 22, 156
U. S. Vitamin & Pharmaceutical Corp., 81, 97

Vacation, see Travel
Vallence-Owens, J., 171, 175
Veterans Administration, 154
Vim equipment, 78, 79, 83, 86
Visual disturbances, 29
Von Hohenheim, T. B., 40
Von Mering, J., 15, 62
Von Noorden, 52

Walpole, H., 37
Watt, R., 51
Weight loss, 29, 34, 35, 87
Weight reduction, 59, 151, 156
Wells, H. G., 37
Western Ontario Medical School, 62
White, P., 163
Willis, T., 40
Yalow, R. S., 175
Yemenite Jews, 25
Young, F. G., 174

Zuelzer, G., 61